Common Medical
Abbreviations

Common Medical Abbreviations ∾

Luís R. DeSousa, M.D., Ph.D.
João S. DeSousa, B.Sc., M.Sc.
Simon P. DeSousa, B.Sc., M.Sc.
Maria C. DeSousa, B.Sc., M.T., M.P.H.

DELMAR

™

THOMSON LEARNING

Africa • Australia • Canada • Denmark • Japan • Mexico • New Zealand • Philippines
Puerto Rico • Singapore • Spain • United Kingdom • United States

Cover Credit: Michael L. Traylor

Delmar Staff
Publisher: David C. Gordon
Sponsoring Editor: Marion Waldman
Project Editor: Mary P. Robinson

Production Coordinator: Jennifer L. Gaines
Art/Design Coordinator: Michael Traylor
Editorial Assistant: Sarah Holle
Production Services: Susan Geraghty

COPYRIGHT © 1995 Delmar, a division of Thomson Learning, Inc. The Thomson Learning™ is a trademark used herein under license.

Printed in the United States of America
5 6 7 8 9 0 XXX 01

For more information, contact Delmar, 3 Columbia Circle, PO Box 15015, Albany, NY 12212-0515; or find us on the World Wide Web at http://www.delmar.com

International Division List

Asia
Thomson Learning
60 Albert Street, #15-01
Albert Complex
Singapore 189969
Tel: 65 336 6411
Fax: 65 336 7411

Australia/New Zealand:
Nelson/Thomson Learning
102 Dodds Street
South Melbourne, Victoria 3205
Australia
Tel: 61 39 685 4111
Fax: 61 39 685 4199

Latin America:
Thomson Learning
Seneca, 53
Colonia Polanco
11560 Mexico D.F. Mexico
Tel: 525-281-2906
Fax: 525-281-2656

Japan:
Thomson Learning
Palaceside Building 5F
1-1-1 Hitotsubashi, Chiyoda-ku
Tokyo 100 0003 Japan
Tel: 813 5218 6544
Fax: 813 5218 6551

UK/Europe/Middle East
Thomson Learning
Berkshire House
168-173 High Holborn
London
WC1V 7AA United Kingdom
Tel: 44 171 497 1422
Fax: 44 171 497 1426

Canada:
Nelson/Thomson Learning
1120 Birchmount Road
Scarborough, Ontario
Canada M1K 5G4
Tel: 416-752-9100
Fax: 416-752-8102

Library of Congress Cataloging-in-Publication Data
Common medical abbreviations/Luis R. DeSousa...(et al.).
    p. cm.
ISBN 0-8273-6643-4
1. Medicine — Abbreviations—Dictionaries. 2. Medicine — Acronyms—Dictionaries.
3. Medicine — Notation—Dictionaries. I. DeSousa. Luis R.
    [DNLM: 1. Medicine—abbreviations.   W 13 C734 1994]
R123.C595   1994
610 . 148—dc20
DNLM/DLC
for Library of Congress   94-26241
                                                       CIP

Preface

For those of us in the medical world, indiscriminate use of abbreviations in our daily parlance and writings has become a necessity. Lacking a universal forum to create these abbreviations has led to misinterpretation and frequent frustration on the part of many reviewers of health records and parlance. This book has been written with non-medical individuals in mind, and every effort has been made to collect the most frequently used abbreviations.

To decipher individually created abbreviations seems a formidable task. Similar abbreviations have different meanings and connotations in different medical specialities and for different individuals in the same medical specialty! They are more the result of habit and extensive use by different individuals and do not follow any specific and established form or order. Thus some may use a specific abbreviation all in capital letters with or without periods, others may use all lowercase letters, and some even may combine capital and lowercase letters. Variations in symbols, Greek, and Latin letters may be used depending on the individual decision or medical specialty.

This collection of abbreviations is arranged in alphabetical order, and the original Latin words are italicized wherever needed. Different meanings of an abbreviation are mentioned as well. Different combinations of capital and lowercase letters are given as in most common use. Please note, in certain instances hyphens are used to show how the abbreviations are derived.

This collection is in no way a complete list of all the abbreviations and their meanings. Every attempt will be made to include newly formed abbreviations in future editions.

Luís R. DeSousa, M.D., Ph.D.

Please send your comments or feedback to the following address:

P.O. Box 19435
Sacramento, California 95819-0435
U.S.A.

Acknowledgements

My gratitude to my wife, Hind, for her support, and to my son, Philip, for inspiring me to work on this book.

Luís R. DeSousa, M.D., Ph.D.

This book is dedicated to our Loving Parents: Joaquim Victorino De Sousa and Ludgera Felicidade Fernandes, who are always treasured in our memories

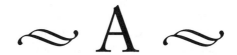

αAAN	alpha-amino acid nitrogen
α_1AT	alpha-one-anti-trypsin
αFP	alpha-feto-protein
αγ G	alpha-gamma-globulinemia
αHBD	alpha-hydroxy-butyric dehydrogenase
αHH	alpha-hydrazine analog of histidine
α_2M	alpha-2 macroglobulin
αMD	alpha-methyl-dopa
αMT	alpha-methyl-tyrosine
αNF	alpha-naphtho-flavone
αNIT	alpha-naphthyl-iso-thiocyanate
αNTU	alpha-naphthyl-thio-urea
AΩA	Alpha Omega Alpha (an honorary society in U.S.A.)
ATγ	anti-thymocyte gamma (globulin)
$\bar{a}$	*ante* (before)
Å	Ångstrom
Ã	cumulated activity
a	*annum* (year); anode; anterior; aorta; *aqua* (water); arabinose; *arteria* (artery); axial
A	absorbance; accommodation; acetum; activity; adenine; adenosine; adult; Adriamycin; age; air; alanine; allergy; alveolar gas; ampere; amphetamine; anesthetic; Angstrom; aqueous; Ara-C; area; argon; Asian; asparaginase; atropine; audio; auricle; average; azote (German word meaning nitrogen); mass number; vitamin A
A_1	aortic first heart sound
A_2	aortic second heart sound
A-1	African variant
AI	angiotensin I
AII	angiotensin II
AIII	angiotensin III
$\bar{a}\ \bar{a}$	so much of each ingredient in a prescription
aa	*arteriae* (arteries)
A&A	aid and attendance; awake and aware
A.A.	Associate in Arts (degree)

AA	acetic acid; achievement age; adenylic acid; African American; Alcoholics Anonymous; alveolar-arterial; amino-acetone; amino-acid; amino-acyl; amyloid A; aortic aneurysm; arachiodonic acid; ascending aorta; Australian antigen; automobile accident
AAA	abdominal aortic aneurysm; acute anxiety attack; amalgam; American Association of Anatomists; aromatic amino acid; atypical adematous adenosis
AAAA	American Academy of Anesthesiologists' Assistants
AAAAPSF	American Association for the Accreditation of Ambulatory Plastic Surgical Facilities
AAAE	amino acid-activating enzymes
AAAF	albumin auto-agglutinating factor
AAAHC	Accreditation Association for Ambulatory Health Care
AA-AMP	amino acid adenylate
aAAN	alpha-amino acid nitrogen
AAAS	American Association for the Advancement of Science
AAATP	Association for Anesthesiologists' Assistants Training Program
AAB	American Association of Bioanalysts
AABB	American Association of Blood Banks
AAC	antibiotic-associated colitis; antimicrobial agents and chemotherapy
AACAHPO	American Association of Certified Allied Health Personnel in Ophthalmology
AACC	American Association for Clinical Chemistry
AACE	American Association of Childbirth Education
AACG	acute angle closure glaucoma
AACIA	American Association for Clinical Immunology and Allergy
AACN	American Association of Colleges of Nursing; American Association of Critical Care Nurses
AACO	American Association of Clinical Oncology
AACP	American Academy of Child Psychiatry
AACR	American Association for Cancer Research
AAD	American Academy of Dermatology
AaDO$_2$	alveolar-arterial oxygen tension difference
AADP	American Academy of Denture Prosthetics
AADR	American Academy of Dental Radiology
AADS	American Association of Dental Schools
AAE	active assisted exercises; acute allergic encephalitis; American Association of Endodontists
AAF	acetic-alcohol-formalin; 2-acetyl-amino-fluorene; ascorbic acid factor

AAFP	American Academy of Family Practice; American Association of Family Physicians
AAGP	American Academy of General Practice
AAH	atypical adenomatous hyperplasia
AAHA	American Academy of Health Administration
AAHC	Association of Academic Health Centers
AAHE	Association for the Advancement of Health Education
AAHP	American Association of Hospital Planners
AAI	American Association of Immunologists; ankle-arm index
AAID	American Academy of Implant Dentistry
AAL	anterior axillary line
AALAS	American Association for Laboratory Animal Science
AAM	American Academy of Microbiology
AAMA	American Association of Medical Assistants
AAMC	American Association of Medical Colleges
AAMD	American Association on Mental Deficiency
AAME	acetyl-arginine methyl ester
AAMI	Association for Advancement of Medical Instrumentation
AAMRL	American Association of Medical Record Librarians
AAMT	American Association for Medical Transcriptionists
AAN	American Academy of Neurology; American Academy of Nursing; analgesic-associated nephropathy
AANA	American Association of Nurse Anesthetists
AANN	American Association of Neuroscience Nurses
AAO	American Academy of Ophthalmology; American Academy of Orthodontists; American Academy of Otolaryngology; amino acid oxidase; awake, alert, oriented
AAOC	ant-acid of choice
AAOP	American Academy of Oral Pathology
AAOS	American Academy of Orthopaedic Surgeons
AAP	air atmospheric pressure; American Academy of Pediatrics; American Academy of Pedodontics; American Academy of Periodontology; American Association of Pathologists
AAPA	American Association of Pathologist Assistants; American Academy of Physician Assistants
AAPB	American Association of Pathologists and Bacteriologists
AAPC	antibiotic-associated pseudomembranous colitis
AAPMR	American Academy of Physical Medicine and Rehabilitation
AAPPO	American Association of Preferred Provider Organizations
AAR	antigen-antiglobulin reaction
AARC	American Association for Respiratory Care

AAROM	active assisted range of motion
AARP	American Association of Retired Persons
AART	American Association for Rehabilitation Therapy; American Association of Respiratory Therapy
AAS	anthrax anti-serum; aortic arch syndrome; atomic absorption spectrophotometry
AASH	adrenal androgen stimulating hormone
a_1AT	alpha-one-anti-trypsin
AAT	alanine amino-transferase; atrium atrium triggered (pacemaker mode); Auditory Acuity Test; Auditory Apperception Test
AATS	American Association for Thoracic Surgery
a.a.u.	*agita ante usum* (shake before using)
AAV	adeno-associated virus; AIDS-associated virus
a.b.	*agita bene* (shake well); *abortus* (abortion)
ab.	*abortio* (abortion)
Ab	anti-body
A.B.	*Artium Baccalaureus* (Bachelor of Arts)
A/B	acid / base (ratio)
A>B	air greater than bone
AB	abnormal; aids to the blind; alcian blue; anti-body; antigen binding; apex beat; asbestos body; asthmatic bronchitis; axio-buccal
ABA	allergic bronchopulmonary aspergillosis; American Board of Anesthesiology; anti-bacterial activity
ABAI	American Board of Allergy and Immunology
ABC	absolute basophil count; acid buffered citrate; Adriamycin, BCNU, Cyclophosphamide; airway, breathing, circulation; American Blood Commission; aneurysmal bone cyst; antigen-binding capacity; apnea, bradycardia, cyanosis; aspiration biopsy cytology; axio-bucco-cervical
ABCD	Adriamycin, Bleomycin, CCNU, Dacarbazine
ABCM	Adriamycin, Bleomycin, Cytoxan, Mitomycin C
ABCP	American Board of Cardiovascular Perfusion
ABCRS	American Board of Colon and Rectal Surgery
ABCW	atomic, biological, and chemical warfare
abd.	abdomen; abdominal; abduct; abduction; abductor
ABD	Adriamycin, Bleomycin, DTIC; aged, blind, disabled
ABDCT	atrial bolus dynamic computer tomography
ABDIC	Adriamycin, Bleomycin, Dimethyl-Imidazole-Carboxamide
abd pain	abdominal pain
abd poll	abductor pollicis

ABDV	Adriamycin, Bleomycin, DTIC, Vinblastine
ABE	acute bacterial endocarditis
ABEM	American Board of Emergency Medicine
ABET	Accreditation Board for Engineering and Technology
ab. feb.	*absente febre* (while fever is absent)
ABFP	American Board of Family Practice
ABG	arterial blood gas; axio-bucco-gingival
ABGs	arterial blood gases
ABI	ankle-brachial index; atherothrombotic brain infarction
ABIM	American Board of Internal Medicine
ABL	abeta-lipoproteinemia; axio-bucco-lingual
ABLB	alternate binaural loudness balance
ABLC	amphotericin B lipid complex
ABMA	anti-basement membrane antibody
ABMM	American Board of Medical Management
ABMS	Advisory Board for Medical Specialties
abn.	abnormal; abnormality
ABNF(HE)	Association of Black Nursing Faculty (in Higher Education)
ABNM	American Board of Nuclear Medicine
abnorm.	abnormal; abnormality
ABNS	American Board of Neurological Surgery
abo.	*abortio* (abortion)
ABO	absent bed occupancy; American Board of Otolaryngology; three main blood types
ABOG	American Board of Obstetrics and Gynecology
abor.	*abortio* (abortion)
ABOS	Adriamycin, Bleomycin, Oncovin, Streptozotocin; American Board of Orthopaedic Surgery
ABP	Adriamycin, Bleomycin, Prednisone; American Board of Pathology; American Board of Pediatrics; androgen-binding protein; antigen-binding protein; arterial blood pressure
ABPA	allergic broncho-pulmonary aspergillosis
ABPANC	American Board of Post Anesthesia Nursing Certification
ABPM	American Board of Preventive Medicine; ambulatory blood pressure monitoring
ABPMR	American Board of Physical Medicine and Rehabilitation
ABMT	allogenic bone marrow transplantation
ABPN	American Board of Psychiatry and Neurology
ABPS	American Board of Plastic Surgery
abr.	abrasions
ABR	abortus-Bang ring (test); absolute bed rest; American Board of Radiology; auditory brain response

abs.	abscess; absent; absolute; absorption
ABS	absent; absolute; absorption; acute brain syndrome; admitting blood sugar; alkyl-benzene sulfonate
abs. fev.	*absente febre* (while fever is absent)
ABSR	auditory brain stem response
abst.	abstract
ABTS	American Board of Thoracic Surgery
ABU	American Board of Urology
ABV	Actinomycin D, Bleomycin, Vincristine; Adriamycin, Bleomycin, Velban
ABVD	Adriamycin, Bleomycin, Vinblastine, Dacarbazine
ABW	actual body weight
ABX	antibiotics
a/c	alternating (electrical) current
a.c.	*ante cibum* (before meals); alternating (electrical) current
Ac	actinium; acetyl; acute
AC	abdominal circumference; acromio-clavicular; adrenal cortex; adreno-corticoid; Adriamycin, Cyclophospha-mide; air-conditioner; air conduction; all cultures; alternating (electrical) current; anodic closure; anterior chamber; anti-cholinergic; anti-coagulant; anti-complementary; aortic closure; atrio-carotid; auri-culocarotid; axio-cervical
AC/A	accommodative convergence / accommodation (ratio)
ACA	accessory conduction-ablation; adeno-carcinoma; American College of Angiology; American College of Apothecaries; anterior cerebral artery; anti-centromere antibody; Automatic Clinical Analyzer
ACAPI	anterior cerebral artery pulsatility index
ACAT	Automatic Computerized Axial Tomography
acb	before breakfast
ACB	antibody-coated bacteria
AC/BC	air conduction / bone conduction
ACBE	air contrast barium enema
acc.	accident; accommodation; according; *accuratissime* (most accurately)
ACC	accumulator; Acute Care Center; adenoid cystic carci-noma; Ambulatory Care Center; American College of Cardiology; anodal closure contraction
AcChS	acetyl-choline-sterase
ACCI	anodal closure clonus
accom.	accommodation
ACCP	American College of Chest Physicians

ACCR	amylase creatinine clearance ratio
ACCT	account; acute cervical cord trauma
accur.	*accuratissime* (most accurately)
ACD	absolute cardiac dullness; acid citrate dextrose; allergic contact dermatitis; American College of Dentists; annihilation coincidence detection; anterior chest diameter
AC/DC	bisexual (slang)
ACD sol.	acid citrate dextrose solution
ACE	acetaminophen; acetone; acetonitrile; acute cerebellar encephalopathy; adrenal cortical extract; Adriamycin, Cytoxan, Etoposide; angiotensin converting enzyme
ACEI	angiotensin converting enzyme inhibitor
ACEP	American College of Emergency Physicians
acetyl-CoA	acetyl-coenzyme A
ACF	accessory clinical findings; acute care facility; anterior cervical fusion
AcFuCy	Actinomycin D, Fluorouracil, Cytoxan
AcG	accelerator globulin (coagulation Factor V)
ACG	American College of Gastroenterology; angio-cardiography; angle closure glaucoma; apex-cardio-gram
ACGME	Accreditation Council for Graduate Medical Education
ACh	acetyl-choline
ACH	adrenal cortical hormone
ACHA	American College of Hospital Administrators
AChE	acetyl-cholin-esterase
AChR	acetyl-choline receptor
AChRab	acetyl-choline receptor anti-body
ac & hs	*ante cibum et hora somni* (before meals and at bed-time)
ACI	acoustic comfort index; adenylate cyclase inhibitor; adrenal cortical insufficiency; anti-clonus index
acid phos.	acid phosphatase
ACIOC	anterior chamber intra-ocular (lens)
ACIP	Advisory Committee on Immunization Practices
ACK	acknowledge
ACL	anterior cruciate ligament; aspiryl chloride
aCLA	anti-cardio-lipin antibody
ACLA	American Clinical Laboratory Association
ACLAM	American College of Laboratory Animal Medicine
ACLS	advanced cardiac life support
ACM	Adriamycin, Cyclophosphamide, Methotrexate; albumin-calcium-magnesium
ACN	acute conditioned necrosis
ACNHA	American College of Nursing Home Administrators

ACNM	American College of Nuclear Medicine; American College of Nurse Midwives
ACO	anodal closure odor
ACOG	American College of Obstetricians and Gynecologists
ACOP	Adriamycin, Cyclophosphamide, Oncovin, Prednisone
ACOPP	Adriamycin, Cytoxan, Oncovin, Prednisone, Procarbazine
ACOS	American College of Osteopathic Surgeons
ACOSPC	American College of Surgeons Pattern of Care
acous.	acoustic
ACP	acid phosphatase; acyl carrier protein; American College of Pathologists; American College of Physicians; Animal Care Panel; anodal closure picture; Aspirin, Caffeine, Phenacetin
ACPE	American College of Physician Executives
ACPP	adreno-cortico-poly-peptide
ACPS	acro-cephalo-poly-syndactyly
ACR	acriflavine; adenomatosis of colon and rectum; American College of Radiology; anti-constipation regimen
acs	before supper
ACS	acute confusional state; Advanced Cardiovascular System; Advanced Catheter System; American Cancer Society; American Chemical Society; American College of Surgeons; American Cytology Society; anodal closing sound; antireticular cytotoxic serum; Association of Clinical Scientists
ACSM	American College of Sports Medicine
ACSV	aorto-coronary saphenous vein
ACT	Actinomycin; activated clotting time; activated coagulation time; active; advanced coronary treatment; anodal closure tetanus; anti-coagulant therapy; axial computed tomography
ACTA	American Cardiovascular Technologists Association; American Corrective Therapy Association; Automated Computerized Transverse Axial
Act-C	Actinomycin C
Act-D	Actinomycin D
ACTe	anodal closure tetanus
ACTG	AIDS Clinic Trial Group
ACTGS	AIDS Clinic Trial Group Study
ACTH	adreno-cortico-tropic hormone
ACTH-RF	adreno-cortico-tropic hormone releasing factor
ACTP	adreno-cortico-tropic polypeptide

ACUTNS	acupuncture / transcutaneous nerve stimulation
ACV	acyclovir; atrial, carotid, ventricular
ACVD	acute cardio-vascular disease
ACVM	American College of Veterinary Microbiologists
ACVP	American College of Veterinary Pathologists
Ad	anisotropic disk
a.d.	*auris dextra* (right ear)
ad	*ad* (indication of something to be added to a certain amount)
A.D.	*anno Domini* (in the year of the Lord)
A/D	analog-to-digital (converter)
A&D	admission and discharge; ascending and descending
AD	accident dispensary; active disease; admitting diagnosis; advertisement; alcohol dehydrogenase; Aleutian disease; Alzheimer's disease; analgesic dose; anodal duration; antigenic determinant; aortic diameter; arthritic dose; autonomic dysreflexia; average deviation; axio-distal; axis deviation
ADA	adenosine-deaminase; American Dental Association; American Diabetic Association; American Dietetic Association; Americans with Disabilities Act; anterior descending artery
ADAA	American Dental Assistants Association
ADAM	animated dissection of anatomy for medicine
ADAMHA	Alcohol, Drug Abuse, and Mental Health Administration
ADB	Adriamycin, Dacarbazine, Bleomycin
ADBC	Adriamycin, DTIC, Bleomycin, CCNU
ADC	Aid to Dependent Children; AIDS Dementia Complex; albumin, dextrose, catalase; analog-to-digital conversion; analog-to-digital converter; anodal duration contraction; average daily census; axio-disto-cervical
ADCC	antibody-dependent cellular cytotoxicity
add.	*adde* (let there be added; add); adding; adduction; adductor
ADD	adduction; attention deficit disorder; average daily dose
ad def. an.	*ad defectionem animi* (to the point of fainting)
ad deliq.	*ad deliquim* (to fainting)
addn	addition
ADDR	address
ade.	adenine
ADE	acute disseminated encephalitis; apparent digestive energy
ad effect.	*ad effectum* (until effectual)

ADEM	acute disseminating encephalo-myelitis
ADG	atrial diastolic gallop; axio-disto-gingival
ad grat. acid.	*ad gratum aciditatem* (to an agreeable sourness)
ADH	acute dehydration; anti-diuretic hormone; alcohol de-hydrogenase
ADHA	American Dental Hygienists Association
ADHD	attention deficit hyperactivity disorder
adhib.	*adhibendus* (to be administered)
ADI	acceptable daily intake; allowable daily intake; axio-disto-incisal
A-DIC	Adriamycin, Dimethyl-Imidazole-Carboxamide
ad int.	*ad interim* (meanwhile)
Adj	adjoining; adjunct; adjustment (bookkeeping abbreviation)
ADL	activities of daily living
ad lib.	*ad libitum* (as desired)
ADM	administrative medicine; admission; admit; admitted
admin.	administer; administration
admov.	*admove* (add); *admoveatur* (let there be added)
adm w/c	admitted in wheel-chair
A.D.N.	Associate Degree in Nursing
ADN	anti-deoxyribo-nuclease
ad neut.	*ad neutro* (neutralize)
ADO	axio-disto-occlusal
AdOAP	Adriamycin, Oncovin, Ara-C, Prednisone
AdOP	Adriamycin, Oncovin, Prednisone
ADP	adenosine-di-phosphate; area diastolic pressure; automatic data processing
ad part. dol.	*ad parte dolente* (to the painful part)
ADPL	average daily patient load
ad pond. om.	*ad pondus omnium* (to the whole weight)
ADR	adverse drug reaction
Adria.	Adriamycin
ADS	antibody deficiency syndrome; anti-diuretic substance
ad sat.	*ad saturatum* (to saturation)
ads. feb.	*adstante febre* (while there is fever)
ADT	adenosine triphosphate; admission, discharge, transfer; agar-gel diffusion test; alternate-day therapy; alternate-day treatment; anodal duration tetanus; atrial demand triggered (pacemaker)
ad us.	*ad usum* (usage)
ad us. ext.	*ad usum externum* (for external use)
a.d.v.	*ad duas vices* (to two doses; for two doses)
adv.	*adversum* (against); advice; advise; advisory

ADV	adeno-virus; advance; advantage; Aleutian disease virus
advan.	advantage; advantages
ADX	adrenalectomized
A/E	air entry
AE	above elbow; air entry; ary-epiglottic
AEA	alcohol, ether, acetone
AE amp.	above elbow amputation
AEC	at earliest convenience; Atomic Energy Commission
AECG	ambulatory ECG
AED	automatic external defibrillator
AEF	allogenic effect factor
aeg.	*aegra* (patient)
AEG	air encephalo-gram
AEI	atrial escape interval
AEM	analytical electron microscope; analytical electron microscopy
AEP	artificial endocrine pancreas; average evoked potential
aeq.	*aequales* (equal)
AER	aldosterone excretion rate; anabolic energy requirements; auditory evoked response; average evoked response
AES	American Electroencephalographic Society
aet.	*aetas* (at the age of)
AET	absorption equivalent thickness; automatic ectopic tachycardia
aetat.	*aetatis* (of the age)
AETB	2-amin-ethyliso-thiuronium bromide
AEV	avian erythroblastosis virus
AF	abnormal frequency; aflatoxin; air-force; albumin-free; amniotic fluid; angiogenesis factor; antibody-forming; aortic flow; atrial fibrillation; atrial flutter; audio frequency
AFA	American Fertility Association
AFB	acid-fast bacillus; acid-fast bacteria; aflatoxin B
AFBG	aorto-femoral bypass graft
AFC	antibody-forming cells
AFCR	American Federation for Clinical Research
AFDC	Aid to Families with Dependent Children
AFG	aflatoxin G
aFGF	acidic fibroblast growth factor
AFH	anterior facial height
AFib	atrial fibrillation
AFID	alkali flame ionization detector
AFL	aflatoxicol; anti-fatty liver; atrial flutter

AFM	aflatoxin M
AFO	ankle-foot orthosis
aFP	alpha-feto-protein
AFP	atrial filling pressure; anterior faucial pillar
AFPP	acute fibrino-purulent pneumonia
AFQ	aflatoxin Q
AFRD	acute febrile respiratory disease
AFS	American Fertility Society
AFSP	acute fibrino-serous pneumonia
AFT	aflatoxin; afternoon
AFTC	apparently free testosterone concentration
AFTN	autonomously functioning thyroid nodule
AFV	amniotic fluid volume
Ag	antigen; *argentum* (silver)
A/G	albumin / globulin (ratio)
AG	abdominal girth; anti-globulin; atrial gallop; axio-gingival
AGA	American Gastroenterological Association; appropriate for gestational age
AGC	automatic gain control
AGE	acute gastroenteritis; agarose gel electrophoresis
AgCl	argentum-chloride (silver chloride)
AGD	agar gel diffusion
AGEPC	acetyl glyceryl ether phosphoryl choline
ag. feb.	*aggrediente febre* (while the fever is coming on)
aGG	alpha-gamma-globulinemia
aggl.	agglutinate; agglutination
AGGS	anti-gas gangrene serum
AgI	argentum-iodide (silver iodide)
agit.	*agita* (shake; stir)
agit. a. s.	*agita ante sumedum* (shake before taking)
agit. vas.	*agitato vase* (shake the vial)
AGL	acute granulocytic leukemia
AGM	African green monkey
AGMK	African green monkey kidney (tissue culture)
AGML	acute gastric mucosal lesion
AGN	acute glomerulo-nephritis
AgNO$_3$	argentum-nitrate (silver nitrate)
AGNOR	silver-staining nucleolar organizer regions
Ag$_2$O	argentum-oxide (silver oxide)
AGP	acid glycoprotein; agar-gel precipitation
AGPT	agar-gel precipitation test
AgS	argentum-sulfadiazine (silver sulfadiazine)
AGS	adreno-genital syndrome

Ag_2SO_4	argentum-sulfate (silver sulfate)
AGT	adreno-glomerulo-tropin; anti-globulin test
AGTT	abnormal glucose tolerance test
AGV	aniline gentian violet
a.h.	*alternis horis* (every other hour)
ah.	hypermetropic astigmatism
Ah	ampere hour
AH	abdominal hysterectomy; accidental hypothermia; aceto-hexamide; amenorrhea and hirsutism; amino-hippurate; anti-hyaluronidase; arterial hypertension; artificial heart; ascites hepatoma
AHA	aceto-hydroxamic acid; acquired hemolytic anemia; American Heart Association; American Hospital Association; aspartyl-hydroxamine acid; autoimmune hemolytic anemia
AHBBP	amino-hydroxy-butylidene bio-phosphate
aHBD	alpha-hydroxy-butyric dehydrogenase
AHC	acute hemorrhagic conjunctivitis; acute hemorrhagic cystitis
AHCPR	Agency for Health Care Policy and Research
AHD	arteriosclerotic heart disease; atherosclerotic heart disease
AHEM	acute hemorrhagic encephalo-myelitis
AHF	acute heart failure; anti-hemophilic factor
AHFS	American Hospital Formulary Service
AHG	aggregated human globulin; anti-hemolytic globulin (factor); anti-hemophilic globulin; anti-human globulin
AHGS	acute herpetic gingival stomatitis
aHH	alpha-hydrazine analog of histidine
AHH	aryl-hydrocarbon hydroxylase
AHI	active hostility index; apnea / hypopnea index
AHIMA	American Health Information Management Association
AHJ	artificial hip joint
AHLE	acute hemorrhagic leuko-encephalitis
AHLS	anti-human lymphocytic serum
AHM	ambulatory Holter monitoring; anterior hyaloid membrane
AHMA	American Holistic Medical Association
AHP	Accountable Health Plan; acute hemorrhagic pancreatitis
AHPA	American Health Planning Association
AHR	autonomic hyper-reflexia
AHS	American Humane Society
AHT	augmented histamine test; anti-hyaluronidase titer
AHTG	anti-human thymocytic globulin

AHuG	aggregated human globulin
AI	anaphylatoxin inhibitor; anatomic index; aortic incompetency; aortic insufficiency; apical impulse; artificial insemination; artificial intelligence; axio-incisal
AIA	allyl-isopropyl-acetamide; amylase inhibitor activity
AIBA	amino-iso-butyric acid
AIC	amino-imidazole carboxamide; anti-inflammatory corticoid
AICA	anterior inferior communicating artery
AICAH	auto-immune chronic active hepatitis (lispoid hepatitis)
AICD	automatic implantable cardiac defibrillator; automatic implantable cardiovascular defibrillator
AICF	auto-immune complement fixation
AID	acute infectious disease; Agency for International Development; artificial insemination by donor (heterologous insemination); auto-immune deficiency; auto-immune disease; automatic implantable defibrillator
AIDS	acquired immuno-deficiency syndrome
AIE	acute infectious encephalitis; acute infective endocarditis
AIEP	amount of insulin extractable from the pancreas
AIF	aorto-ilio-femoral
AIGO	amyloid of immuno-globulin origin
AIH	American Institute of Homeopathy; artificial insemination by husband (homologous insemination)
AIHA	American Industrial Hygiene Association; auto-immune hemolytic anemia
AIHD	acquired immune hemolytic disease; auto-immune hemolytic disease
AILD	angio-immunoblastic lymphadenopathy with dysproteinemia
AIM	assess, improve, maintain
AIMS	abnormal involuntary movement scale
AIN	acute interstitial nephritis
AINS	anti-inflammatory non-steroidal
AIO	amyloid of immunoglobulin origin
AIP	acute intermittent porphyria; automated immunoprecipitation; average intravascular pressure
AIPL	angiocentric immuno-proliferative lesions
AIR	amino-imidazole ribonucleotide
AIS	anti-insulin serum; androgen insensitivity syndrome
AIT	alanine amino-transferase

AITP	auto-immune thrombocytopenic purpura
AITT	arginine insulin tolerance test
AIU	absolute iodine uptake
AIUM	American Institute of Ultrasound in Medicine
AIVR	accelerated idio-ventricular rhythm
AJ	ankle jerk
AJCC	American Joint Committee on Cancer
AK	above knee; adenylate kinase; atrial kick
AKA	above knee amputation; alcoholic keto-acidosis; also known as
Al	aluminum (used in U.S.A); aluminium (used in U.K.)
AL	active lipid; acute leukemia; adaptation level; albumin; alcohol; auris laeva; axio-lingual
ALA	Active Labor Act; alanine; American Lung Association; amino-levulinic acid; axio-labial
ALAD	abnormal left axis deviation; amino-levulinic acid dehydratase
ALAG	axio-labio-gingival
ALAL	axio-labio-lingual
ALAT	alanine transaminase
alb.	*albus* (albumin)
ALB	alternate loudness balance
ALC	alcohol; alcoholic; axio-linguo-cervical; approximate lethal concentration; avian leukosis complex
ALD	adreno-leuko-dystrophy; alcoholic liver disease; aldolase; angioimmunoblastic lympha-denopathy
ALG	anti-lymphocytic globulin; axio-linguo-gingival
alk.	alkaline
alk. phos.	alkaline phosphatase
ALL	acute lymphatic leukemia; acute lymphoblastic leukemia; acute lymphocytic leukemia; allergies; allergy; allose axio-labio-lingual
ALM	acral lentiginous melanoma; alveolar lining material
ALME	acetyl-lysine methyl ester
ALMI	antero-lateral myocardial infarction
ALN	anterior lymph node
ALO	axio-linguo-occlusal
Al_2O_3	aluminum-oxide (aluminium-oxide)
$Al(OH)_3$	aluminum-hydroxide (aluminium-hydroxide)
ALOMAD	Adriamycin, Leukeran, Oncovin, Methotrexate, Actinomycin D, Dacarbazine
ALOS	average length of stay

ALP	alkaline phosphatase; alkyl lyso-phospholipids; anterior lobe of pituitary; anti-lymphocyte plasma
ALPS	Aphasia Languages Performance Scales
ALRI	antero-lateral rotary instability
ALRR	arthroscopic lateral retinacular release
ALS	acute lateral sclerosis; advanced life support; alternating chemotherapy with radiotherapy without delay of chemotherapy; amyotrophic lateral sclerosis; angiotensin-like substance; antero-lateral sclerosis; anticipated life span; anti-lymphatic serum; anti-lymphocyte serum
alt.	*alter* (the other); alternate; altitude
ALT	alanine amino-transferase; alanine transaminase (formerly SGPT); argon laser trabeculoplasty
ALT/AST	alanine amino-transferase / aspartate amino-transferase (ratio)
ALTB	acute laryngo-tracheo-bronchitis
alt. dieb	*alternis diebus* (every other day)
alt. hor.	*alternis horis* (every other hour)
alt. noc.	*alternis nocte* (every other night)
ALT-RCC	auto-lymphocyte-based treatment for renal cell carcinoma
ALU	arithmetic and logic unit (in a computing processor)
ALV	alveolar; avian leukosis virus
alv. adst.	*alvo adstricta* (when the bowels are constipated)
ALW	arch-loop-whorl system
a.m.	*anno mundi* (in the year of the world); *ante meridiem* (being before noon); *ante mortem* (preceding death)
a$_2$M	alpha-2 macroglobulin
Am	Americium
AM	actomyosin; aerospace medicine; alveolar macrophage; American; ametropia; ampicillin; amplitude modulation; anovular menstruation; arousal mechanism; *Artium Magister* (Master of Arts); aviation medicine; axiomesial; before noon; myopic astigmatism
AMA	against medical advice; American Medical Association; anti-mitochondrial antibody; as much as
AMACT	anti-microbial agents and chemo-therapy
AMA-ERF	AMA — Education and Research Foundation
AMA-Fab	antimyosin monoclonal antibody with Fab fragment
AMAP	as much as possible
AMB	ambiguous; ambulance; ambulate; ambulatory
AMBL	acute mono-blastic leukemia
AMC	arm muscle circumference; arthrogryposis multiplex congenita; axio-mesio-cervical

AMCL	acute mono-cytic leukemia
aMD	alpha-methyl-dopa
AMD	arthroscopic micro-diskectomy; axio-mesio-distal
AME	amphotericin methyl ester
AMEA	American Medical Electroencephalographic Association
Amerind.	American Indian
AMF	amniotic fluid; anti-muscle factor
AmFAR	American Foundation for AIDS Research
AMG	anti-macrophage globulin; axio-mesio-gingival
AMH	mixed astigmatism with myopia predominating
AMI	acute myocardial infarction; American Indian; amitriptyline; anterior myocardial infarction; Association of Medical Illustrators; axio-mesio-incisal
AMKBL	acute mega-karyo-blastic leukemia
AML	acute monocytic leukemia; acute myeloblastic leukemia; acute myelocytic leukemia; acute myelogenous leukemia; acute myeloid leukemia; anterior mitral leaflet
AMLP	anatomic medullary locking prosthesis
AMLR	autologus mixed lymphocyte reaction
AMLS	anti-mouse lymphocyte serum
AMM	agnogenic myeloid metaplasia; ammonia
AMMBL	acute myelo-mono-blastic leukemia; acute myelo-mono-blastic lymphoma
AMMCL	acute myelo-mono-cytic leukemia
AMN	alloxazine mono-nucleotide; American Medical News
AMO	axio-mesio-occlusal
A-mode	amplitude mode
amp.	ampere; amphetamine; ampicillin; ampule; amputation
AMP	acid muco-polysaccharide; adenosine mono-phosphate; amplifier; amplitude; average mean pressure; Rifampin
AMPAC	American Medical Political Action Committee
AMPase	adenosine mono-phosphat-ase
amph.	amphetamine; amphoric
AMP kinase	adenylate kinase
ampl.	amplitude; *amplus* (large)
AMPPE	acute multifocal placoid pigment epitheliopathy
AMPS	abnormal muco-poly-sacchariduria; acid muco-poly-saccharides
AMRA	American Medical Record Association
AMRD	Anti-microbial Removal Device
AMRI	ametro-medial rotatory instability
AMRL	Aerospace Medical Research Laboratories

AMS	acute mountain sickness; amylase; anti-macrophage serum; Army Medical Service; atypical measles syndrome; auditory memory span; automated multiphasic screening
amsa.	amsacrine
AMSA	acridinylaniside; American Medical Students Association
amt.	amount
aMT	alpha-methyl-tyrosine
AMT	American Medical Technologists; amethopterin; amphetamine; amount
amu	atomic mass unit
AMV	assisted mechanical ventilation
AMWA	American Medical Women's Association; American Medical Writers Association
amy.	amylase
AMZ	antero-medial displacement osteotomy
an.	anode
An	Actinon; anisometropia; anodal; anode
A/N	as needed
AN	aneurysm; anorexia nervosa; ante-natal; aseptic necrosis; avascular necrosis
ana	so much of each
ANA	American Nurses Association; anti-nuclear antibody; aspartyl naphthyl-amide
ANAC	Association of Nurses in AIDS Care
anal.	analgesia; analgesic
ANAP	agglutination negative, absorption positive
anat.	anatomic; anatomical; anatomy
ANC	absolute neutrophil count
AnCC	anodal closure contraction
ANDA	abbreviated new drug application
andro.	androsterone
AnDTe	anodal duration tetanus
anes.	anesthesia; anesthetic
aNF	alpha-naphtho-flavone
ANF	American Nurses Foundation; anti-nuclear factor; atrial natriuretic factor
ang.	angiogram; angiograph; angle
angio.	angiocatheter; angiocatheterizaton; angiography
ANHB	Alaska Native Health Board
anhyd.	anhydrous
ANISO	anisocytosis; anisometropia
aNIT	alpha-naphthyl-iso-thiocyanate
ank.	ankle

ANLL	acute non-lymphoblastic leukemia; acute non-lympho-cytic leukemia
annl.	annual; annulatomy; annulorrhaphy
ANP	A-nor-progesterone; atrial natriuretic polypeptide
ANRC	American National Red Cross
ANS	answer; anterior nasal spine; anti-neutrophilic serum; arteriolo-nephro-sclerosis; autonomic nervous system
ANSA	amino-naphthol-sulfonic acid
ANSI	American National Standards Institute
ant.	*ante* (before)
ANT	acoustic noise test; anterior; anthropology
Ant. A	Antamycin A
antag.	antagonistic
ant ax line	anterior axillary line
anthrop.	anthropology
anti-AChR	anti-acetyl-choline receptor
anti-coag	anti-coagulant
anti-DNA	anti-deoxyribo-nucleic acid
anti-FY	Duffy antibody
anti-GBM	anti-glomerular basement membrane
anti-HAA	antibody to hepatitis-associated antigen
anti-HAV	anti-hepatitis A virus
anti-HB	anti-hepatitis B
anti-HBC	antibody to hepatitis B core antigen
anti-HBS	antibody to hepatitis B surface antigen
anti-HLTD III	antibody screen in testing for AIDS
anti-S	anti-sulfanilic acid
anti-T$_3$	triiodothyronine auto-antibodies
ant. part.	*ante partum* (before delivery)
ant. pit.	anterior pituitary
ant. pran.	*ante prandium* (before dinner)
ant. tib.	anterior tibial
aNTU	alpha-naphthyl-thio-urea
ANUG	acute necrotizing ulcerative gingivitis
a/o	angle of
A-O	acoustic-optic; awake and oriented
A&O	awake and oriented
AO	acid output; acridine orange; anodal opening; anterior oblique; aortic opening; atomic orbital; atrioventricular opening (of the valves); axio-occlusal
AOA	Alpha Omega Alpha (an honorary society in U.S.A.); American Optometric Association; American Orthopsychiatric Association; American Osteopathic Association

AOAA	amino-oxy-acetic acid
AOB	accessory olfactory bulb; alcohol on breath
AOC	abridged ocular chart; anodal opening clonus; anodal opening contraction
AOD	arterial occlusive disease; auriculo-osteo-dysplasia
AODM	adult onset diabetes mellitus
AOIVM	angiographically occult intracranial vascular malformation
AOL	acro-osteo-lysis
AOM	acute otitis media; alternatives of management
AOMA	American Occupational Medical Association
AONE	American Organization of Nurse Executives
AOO	anodal opening odor
AoP	left ventricle to aorta pressure gradient
AOP	anodal opening picture; aortic pressure
AOPA	American Orthotics and Prosthetics Association
AOR	Alvarado Orthopedic Research
AORN	Association of Operating Room Nurses
AOS	anodal opening sound
AOSSM	American Orthopaedic Society for Sports Medicine
AOTA	American Occupational Therapy Association
AOTe	anodal opening tetanus
AOU	apparent oxygen utilization
AOV	analysis of variance
Ap.	April
A&P	anterior and posterior; auscultation and palpation; auscultation and percussion
AP	acid phosphatase; action potential; acute proliferative; alkaline phosphatase; amino-peptidase; angina pectoris; ante partum; anterior pituitary; antero-posterior; aortic pressure; apical pulse; apriori (prior to); arterial pressure; atrial pacing; atrium pacing; axio-pulpal
APA	aldosterone-producing adenoma; American Pharmaceutical Association; American Physiotherapy Association; American Podiatric Association; American Psychiatric Association; American Psychological Association; amino-penicillanic acid; anti-pernicious anemia (factor)
APACHE	acute physiology and chronic health evaluation
APAP	Acetaminophen (Acamol; Calpol; Dirox; Dymadon; Tylenols); Association of Physician Assistants Programs
APAS	annular phased array system
APB	abductor pollicis brevis; atrial premature beat
APC	adenoid-pharyngeal-conjunctival; Amsacrine, Prednisone, Chlorambucil; anti-phlogistic corticoid;

	antigen-presenting cell; Aspirin, Phenacetin, Caffeine; atrial premature complex; atrial premature contraction
APC-C	Aspirin, Phenacetin, Caffeine with Codeine
APCD	adult polycystic (kidney) disease
APCF	acute pharyngo-conjunctival fever
APD	antero-posterior diameter; atrial premature depolarization
APE	acetone powder extract; acute psychotic episode; acute pulmonary edema; Aminophylline, Phenobarbital, Ephedrine; anterior pituitary extract
APF	anabolism-promoting factor; animal protein factor
APG	acid-precipitable globulin
APGAR	adaptability, partnership, growth, affection, resolve
APH	adenohypo-physeal hormone; ante-partum hemorrhage; anterior pituitary hormone
APHA	American Public Health Association
APhAs	American Pharmaceutical Association
APHP	anti-*Pseudomonas* human plasma
APKD	adult polycystic kidney disease
APL	abductor pollicis longus; accelerated painless labor; acute promyelocytic leukemia; anterior pituitary-like (hormone)
AP-Lat	antero-posterior and lateral
APM	anterior papillary muscle
APMD	automated percutaneous micro-diskectomy
APML	acute pro-myelocytic leukemia
APN	acute pyelo-nephritis; average peak noise
a.p.o.	*ad pondus omnium* (to the weight of the whole)
APO	Adriamycin, Prednisone, Oncovin
apo C	apolipoprotein C
apo D	apolipoprotein D
apo E	apolipoprotein E
app.	*applantus* (flat)
APP	alum-precipitated protein; alum-precipitated pyridine; apparent; appendix; auscultation, percussion, palpation
AP:PA	antero-posterior : postero-anterior
APPG	aqueous procaine penicillin G
applic.	*applicandus* (to be administered)
approx.	approximate; approximately; approximation
appt.	appointment
Apr.	April
APR	abdominal-perineal resection; amebic prevalence rate; anatomic porous replacement; anterior pituitary reaction; April

APRP	acute phase reactant protein
APRT	adenine phospho-ribosyl transferase
APS	adenosine phospho-sulfate; American Physiological Society
APSAC	anisoylated plasminogen streptokinase activator complex
APT	alum-precipitated toxoid; artificial pneumo-thorax; atrial paroxysmal tachycardia; automatic programmed tools
APTA	American Physical Therapy Association
APTT	activated partial thromboplastin time
APT test	aluminum (aluminium) precipitated toxoid test
APUD	amine precursor uptake and decarboxylation
APUD-C	amine precursor uptake and decarboxylation cells
APUD-T	amine precursor uptake and decarboxylation tumors
aq.	*aqua* (water); *aqueus* (water)
AQ	abstraction quotient; accomplishment quotient; achievement quotient; any quantity
aq. bul.	*aqua bulliens* (boiling water)
aq. calc.	*aqua calcariae* (lime water)
aq. calid.	*aqua calida* (warm water)
aq. cam.	*aqua camphorae* (camphor water)
aq. chlori	*aqua chlori* (chlorine water)
aq. dest.	*aqua destillata* (distilled water)
aq. ferv.	*aqua fervens* (hot water)
aq. font.	*aqua fontana* (fountain water); *aqua fontis* (spring water)
aq. fortis	*aqua fortis* (strong water; weak nitric water)
aq. frig.	*aqua frigida* (cold water; frigid water)
aq. m. p.	*aqua menthae piperitae* (peppermint water)
aq. pura	*aqua pura* (pure water)
aq. purif.	*aqua purificata* (purified water)
aq. tepid	*aqua tepida* (tepid water)
Ar	Argon
A/R	apical / radial
A&R	advised and released
AR	achievement ratio; active resistance; alarm reaction; allergic reaction; allergic rhinitis; analytical reagent; androgen receptor; aortic regurgitation; Argyll Robertson (pupil); artificial respiration; atrial rate; auto-radiography
ARA	American Rheumatism Association
Ara-A	Arabinoside-Adenine
Ara-C	Arabinoside-Cytosine
ARAD	abnormal right axis deviation
ARAS	ascending reticular activation system

Ara-U	Arabinosyl-Uracil
ARBOR	arthropod-borne (virus)
ARBP	apo-retinol binding protein
ARC	abnormal retinal correspondence; accelerating rate calorimeter; AIDS-Related Complex; American Red Cross; anamalous retinal correspondence
ARCA	acquired red cell aplasia; American Rehabilitation Counselling Association
ARD	acute respiratory disease; acute respiratory distress; adult respiratory disease; AIDS-Related Disease; Antimicrobial Removal Device; arthritis and rheumatic diseases
ARDS	acute respiratory distress syndrome; adult respiratory distress syndrome
ARF	acute renal failure; acute respiratory failure; acute rheumatic fever; audio response frequency
arg.	*argentum* (silver)
Arg.	arginine; arginyl
ARG	auto-radio-graphy
ARI	airway reactivity index
ARIA	automated radio-immuno-assay
ARL	average remaining lifetime
ARLD	alcohol-related liver disease
ARM	allergy relief medicine; artificial rupture of membrane
ARMD	age-related macular degeneration
ARMs	artificial rupture of membranes
AROA	autosomal recessive ocular albinism
AROM	active range of motion; artificial rupture of membrane(s)
ARP	absolute refractory period; at-risk period
ARROM	active resistive range of motion
ARRS	American Roentgen Ray Society
ARRT	American Registry of Radiologic Technologists
ARS	AIDS-Related Syndrome; anti-rabies serum
ARSM	acute respiratory system malfunction
ART	absolute retention time; Accredited Record Technician; AIDS Resources Team; Automated Reagin Test; artery; arterial; artificial; articulation
ARV	AIDS-Related Virus; anterior right ventricular
ARVO	Association for Research in Vision and Ophthalmology
a.s.	*auris sinistra* (left ear)
A-s	ampere second
As	Arsenic; astigmatic; astigmatism; standard atmosphere

AS	Adam-Stokes (disease); alveolar sac; androsterone sulfate; Anglo-Saxon; ankylosing spondylitis; anti-streptolysin; anxiety state; aortic sounds; aortic stenosis; aqueous solution; arterio-sclerosis; artificial sweetener; astigmatism; athero-sclerosis; audiogenic seizure
ASA	Acetyl Salicylic Acid (Aspirin); Adams-Stokes Attack; American Society of Anesthesiologists; American Standards Association; American Surgical Association; arginino-succinic acid; aryl-sulfatase A; as soon as
ASAHP	American Society of Allied Health Professionals
ASAI	aortic stenosis and aortic insufficiency
ASAP	as soon as possible
ASAS	American Society of Abdominal Surgeons
ASAT	aspartate amino-transferase (formerly SGOT); aspartate transaminase
asb.	asbestiform; asbestos; asbestosis
ASB	American Society of Bacteriologists
ASC	altered state of consciousness; ambulatory surgical center
ASCAD	arterio-sclerotic coronary artery disease
ASCH	American Society of Clinical Hypnosis
ASCII	American Standard Code for Information Interchange
ASCLT	American Society of Clinical Laboratory Technicians
ASCO	American Society of Clinical Oncology; American Society of Contemporary Ophthalmology
ASCP	American Society of Clinical Pathologists
ASCVD	arterio-sclerotic cardio-vascular disease; atherio-sclerotic cardio-vascular disease
ASCVRD	arterio-sclerotic cardio-vascular renal disease
ASD	aldosterone secretion defect; atrial septal defect
ASDC	American Society of Dentistry for Children
ASDH	acute sub-dural hematoma
ASE	American Society of Echocardiography; axilla, shoulder, elbow
ASEP	American Society for Experimental Pathology
ASF	aniline, sulfur, formaldehyde
ASG	anti-serum globulin
ASGE	American Society of Gastrointestinal Endoscopy
ASH	American Society for Hematology; anti-streptococcal hyaluronidase; asymmetrical septal hypertrophy
ASHA	American School Health Association; American Speech and Hearing Association
ASHD	arterio-sclerotic heart disease; athero-sclerotic heart disease

ASHP	American Society of Hospital Pharmacists
ASIF	American Society of Internal Fixation
ASII	American Science Information Institute
ASIM	American Society of Internal Medicine
ASIS	anterior superior iliac spines
ASK	anti-strepto-kinase
ASL	American Sign Language; anti-strepto-lysin; arginino-succinate-lyase
ASLC	acute, self-limited colitis
ASLO	anti-strepto-lysin O
ASM	American Society for Microbiology; myopic astigmatism
ASMI	antero-septal myocardial infarct
ASMT	American Society for Medical Technology
ASN	alkali-soluble nitrogen
ASO	anti-streptolysin O; arteriosclerosis obliterans
As_2O_3	arsenic trioxide
ASP	American Society of Parasitologists; asparaginase; asparagine; asparaginyl; aspartic acid; aspartyl
ASPAN	American Society of Post Anesthesia Nurses
ASPET	American Society for Pharmacology and Experimental Therapeutics
ASPS	alveolar soft part sarcoma
ASPVD	arterio-sclerotic peripheral vascular disease
ASR	aldosterone secretion rate; aldosterone secretory rate
ASRT	American Society of Radiologic Technologists
ASS	anterior superior spine; arginino-succinate synthetase
ASSN	association
ASST	assistant
AST	angiotensin sensitivity test; aspartate amino-transferase (formerly SGOT); aspartate transaminase; Association of Surgical Technologists; astigmatism; Atlantic Standard Time
astigm.	astigmatism
ASTO	anti-streptolysin O
as tol.	as tolerated
ASTR	American Society for Therapeutic Radiology
ASTZ	anti-strepto-zyme
ASUTS	American Society of Ultrasound Technical Specialists
ASV	anti-snake venom; arterio-superficial venous
ASVD	arterio-sclerotic vascular disease; athero-sclerotic vascular disease
ASVG	autologous saphenous vein graft
ASVIP	Atrial Synchronous Ventricular Inhibited Pacemaker

asym.	asymmetrical; asymptomatic
At	Astatine
AT	achievement test; Achilles tendon; adenine and thymine; adjunctive therapy; air temperature; Alt Tuberculin (German: old Tuberculin); ami-triptyline; amino-transferase; anaphyla-toxin; anti-thrombin; anti-trypsin; applanation tonometry; arrival time; artificial teeth; artificial tooth; atomic; atrial tachycardia
AT-III	anti-thrombin III
ATA	alimentary toxic aleukia; anti-thyroglobulin antibody; anti-*Toxoplasma* antibodies; atmosphere absolute
atax.	ataxaphasia; ataxia; ataxiagram; ataxiagraph; ataxiameter; ataxiophobia; ataxophemia; ataxphemia
ATC	activated thymus cell; around the clock; atrial tachy-cardia
ATCC	American Type Culture Collection
ATD	Alzheimer-Type Dementia; anti-thyroid drugs; asphyxiating thoracic dystrophy
ATE	adipose tissue extract
ATF	Alcohol, Tobacco and Firearms (Bureau); BATF
ATG	Adenine, Thymine, Guanine; anti-thymocyte globulin; anti-thyro-globulin; antihuman thymocyte globulin
ATGam	anti-thymocyte gamma (globulin)
ATge	gas exchange anaerobic threshold
ATI	abdominal trauma index
ATL	Achilles tendon lengthening; adult T-cell leukemia; adult T-cell lymphoma; atypical lymphocytes
ATLA	adult T-cell leukemia antigen
ATLL	adult T-cell leukemia-lymphoma
ATLS	advanced trauma life support
ATLV	adult T-cell leukemia virus
atm.	atmosphere; atmospheric
ATN	acute tubular necrosis
at. no.	atomic number
ATNR	asymmetric tonic neck reflex
ATP	adenosine tri-phosphate
ATPase	adenosine tri-phosphat-ase
ATPS	ambient temperature and pressure saturated
ATR	Achilles tendon reflex
ATRT	Achilles Tendon Reflex Test
ATS	American Thoracic Society; anti-tetanic serum; anti-thymocyte serum; anxiety tension state
ATT	arginine tolerance test

ATTN	attention
a.t.v.	*ad tertium vicem* (for three doses; three times)
at. wt.	atomic weight
ATZ	anal transition zone; atypical transformation zone
a.u.	*auris uterque* (each ear)
a.u.	*aures unitas* (both ears together)
au.	*aut* (or)
Au	*aurum* (gold)
Å.U	Ångstrom unit
A.U	Angstrom unit
A.U.	antitoxin units; arbitrary units; aza-uridine
AUA	American Urological Association
AuAg	Australian antigen
AuBMT	Autologous Bone Marrow Transplantation
AUC	area under the curve
AUD	*auditiorius* (auditory)
Aug.	August
AUG	acute ulcerative gingivitis; August
AuHAA	Australian hepatitis-associated antigen
AUL	acute undifferentiated leukemia
AUO	amyloid of unknown origin
a.u.p.	*ad usum proprium* (according to proper use)
aur.	*auris* (ear); *aurum* (gold)
aur. fib.	auricular fibrillation
ausc.	auscultation
AuSH	Australian Serum Hepatitis
aut	*aut* (or)
auto.	automobile
Av	average; avoirdupois
A-V	arterio-venous; atrio-ventricular
AV	Adriamycin, Vincristine; alveolar duct; anterior ventral; ant-virin; aortic valve; Arginine, Vasopressin; arterio-venous; artificial ventilation; atrio-ventricular; auricular ventricular node; average
AVB	atrio-ventricular block; atrio-ventricular bundle
AV block	atrio-ventricular block
AVC	allantoin vaginal cream; associative visual cortex; atrio-ventricular canal; atrio-ventricularis communis
AVCD	atrio-ventricular cushion defect
AVCS	atrio-ventricular conduction system
AVD	aortic valve disease; arterio-venous difference
AVDO$_2$	arterio-venous oxygen difference
AVE	aortic valve electrocardiogram

AVECG	aortic valve electro-cardio-gram
AVF	anti-viral factor; arterio-venous fistula
AVH	acute viral hepatitis
AVHB	atrio-ventricular heart block
AVI	acute viral index
AVM	atrio-ventricular malformation; arterio-venous malfunction
AVMA	American Veterinary Medical Association
AVN	atrio-ventricular node; avascular necrosis
AVO	atrio-ventricular opening (of the valves)
AVp	Arginine, Vasopressin
AVP	Actinomycin D, Vincristine, Platinol; anti-viral protein
AVR	aortic valve replacement
AVRP	atrio-ventricular refractory period
AVS	arterio-venous shunt
AVSD	atrio-ventricular septal defect
AVT	Allen Vision Test; Area Ventralis of Tsai; arginine vaso-tocin
AVV	atrio-ventricular valves
A/W	in accordance with
A&W	alive and well
AW	above waist; air-way; air-ways; anterior wall; atomic weight
awa	as well as
AWD	alive with disease
AWF	adrenal weight factor
AWI	anterior wall infarction
AWMI	anterior wall myocardial infarction
AWP	air-way pressure
AWRS	anti-whole rabbit serum
ax.	axial; axilla; axillary; axis
axo.	axometer; axonotmesis
AYF	anti-yeast factor
AYP	autolyzed yeast protein
Az	Azote (nitrogen)
Aza	Azathioprine
AZBQ	Aziridinyl-benzo-quinone
Azg	Azaguanine
AZT	Aschheim-Zondek Test; azido-thymidine

～ B ～

βGP	beta-glycero-phosphatase
βHBA	beta-hydroxy-butyric acid
βHCG	beta-human chorionic gonadotrophin (hormone); pregnancy test (using blood sample)
βHS	beta-hemolytic streptococcus
βLG	beta-lactoglobulin
β_2MG	beta-two-micro-globulin
βOBA	beta-oxy-butyric acid
βPL	beta-propio-lactone
βTMG	beta-2-micro-globulin
BγG	bovine gamma globulin
Ⓑ	both
b.	*balneum* (bath); base; *bis* (twice)
B√	billing information posted
B	baby; bacillus; bad; bag; balantidium; barometric; base; bath; behavior; bell; Bible; big; bicuspid; black; Bleomycin; blind; blond; blood; blue; body; born; boron; boy; brother; Brucella; buccal; magnetic induction; vitamin B
Ba	Barium
B.A.	*Artium Baccalaureus* (Bachelor of Arts)
B>A	bone greater than air
BA	back-ache; bacterial agglutination; betamethasone acetate; blocking antibody; bone age; bovine albumin; brachial artery; bronchial asthma
Bab.	Babinski
BAC	bacterin; blood alcohol concentration; bronchioloalveolar adeno-carcinoma; bucco-axio-cervical; Bunsen absorption coefficient
BACOD	Bleomycin, Adriamycin, CCNU, Oncovin, Dexamethasone
BACON	Bleomycin, Adriamycin, CCNU, Oncovin, Nitrogen-mustard
BACOP	Bleomycin, Adriamycin, Cytoxan, Oncovin, Prednisone

BACT	bacteria; Bacterium; BCNU, Ara-C, Cytoxan, 6-Thioguanine
BAD	biological aerosol detector (ecology); bipolar affective disorder (psychiatric)
BaE	Barium enema
BAEE	benzoyl-arginine ethyl ester; benzyl-arginine ethyl ester
BAG	bucco-axio-gingival
bal.	*balneum* (bath); balance
BAL	balance; blood alcohol level; British anti-lewisite; broncho-alveolar lavage; dimercaprol
BALB	binaural alternate loudness balance (test)
BALF	broncho-alveolar lavage fluid
Bal. fwd.	balance forward (bookkeeping abbreviation)
B-ALL	B-cell acute lymphoblastic leukemia
bal. sin.	*balneum sinapis* (mustard bath)
BALT	bronchus-associated lymphoid tissue
BaM	Barium meal
BAME	benzoyl-arginine methyl ester
BAMON	Bleomycin, Adriamycin, Methotrexate, Oncovin, Nitrogen-mustard
bands	banded neutrophils
BAO	basal acid output
BAO/PAO	basal acid output / peak acid output (ratio)
BAP	blood agar plate
BAPP	Bleomycin, Adriamycin, Platinol, Prednisone
BAPS	biomechanical ankle platform system
BART	blood-activated recalcification time
BAS	British Anatomical Society
BASDLB	block in the antero-superior division of the left branch
BASH	body acceleration given synchronously with the heartbeat
$BaSO_4$	Barium sulfate
basos	basophils
BAT	brain adjacent to tumor; brown adipose tissue
BATF	Bureau of Alcohol, Tobacco and Firearms; ATF
Baudel. M	Baudelocque's Method
BAVIP	Bleomycin, Adriamycin, Velban, Imidazole, Prednisone
BAVP	balloon aortic valvulo-plasty
BB	bed bath; blanket bath; blood bank; blue bloaters; both bones; breast biopsy; buffer base
BBA	born before arrival
BBB	blood-brain barrier; bundle branch block
BBBB	bilateral bundle branch block

BBD	benign breast disease
BBL	bird-breeder's lung
BBR	bundle branch reentry
BBSO	black braided silk out
BBSS	black braided silk suture
BBT	basal body temperature
B&C	bed and chair
BC	bactericidal concentration; birth control; blood culture; bone conduction; Bowman's Capsule; bucco-cervical
BCA	balloon catheter angioplasty
BCAA	branched-chain amino acid
BCAF	basophil chemotaxis augmentation factor
BCAP	balloon catheter angio-plasty
BCAVe	Bleomycin, CCNU, Adriamycin, Velban
BCB	brilliant cresyl blue
BCBR	bilateral carotid body resection
BCC	basal cell carcinoma; birth control clinic
BCD	binary coded decimal; Bleomycin, Cytoxan, Dactinomycin
BCDF	B-cell differentiation factor
BCE	basal cell epithelioma
B-cell	B lymphocyte
BCF	basophil chemotactic factor
BCG	bacillus Calmette-Guérin (vaccine); ballisto-cardio-gram; ballisto-cardio-graph; bi-color guaiac (test); brom-cresol green
BCGF	B-cell growth factor
BCHOP	Bleomycin, Cytoxan, Hydroxydaunomycin, Oncovin, Prednisone
BCL	basic cycle length
B-CLL	B-cell chronic lymphatic leukemia
BCLS	Basic Cardiac Life Support
BCLT	blood clot lysis time
BCM	birth control medication; body cell mass
BCNS	basal cell nevus syndrome (*naevus* = birthmark)
BCNU	bacterially controlled nursing unit; bis-chloroethyl-nitroso-urea (carmustine)
BCOP	BCNU, Cyclophosphamide, Oncovin, Prednisone
BCP	basic calcium phosphate; BCNU, Cytoxan, Prednisone; birth control pills
BCS	Battered Child Syndrome
BCVA	best corrected visual acuity
BCVP	BCNU, Cytoxan, Velban, Procarbazine

BCVPP	BCNU, Cytoxan, Velban, Procarbazine, Prednisone
b.d.	*bis die* (twice a day)
BD	base deficit; bile duct; brain death; bucco-distal; Bucky diaphragm
BDA	Boston Diagnostic Aphasia; British Dental Association
BDC	blue-dome cyst; brain-damaged child; burn-dressing change
BDCL	basic drive-cycle length
BDG	buffered deoxycholate glucose
BD-M	Byrd-Dew method
B-DOPA	Bleomycin, DTIC, Oncovin, Prednisone, Adriamycin
b.d.s.	*bis die sumendum* (to be taken twice a day)
BDS	blue-diaper syndrome; British Dental Society
B.D.Sc.	Bachelor of Dental Science
BDU	bromo-deoxy-uridine
Bé	Baumé
Be	Beryllium
BE	bacillary emulsion; bacterial endocarditis; Barium enema; base excess; below elbow; bovine enteritis
BEAM	BCNU, Etoposide, Ara-C, Melphalan; brain electrical activity map
BE amp.	below elbow amputation
BEC	bacterial endo-carditis; blood ethanol concentration
BEE	basal energy expenditure
bef.	before
beg.	begin; beginning
BEI	butanol-extractable iodine
bene	*bene* (well)
BEP	Bleomycin, Etoposide, Platinol
beri.	beriberi
BES	balanced electrolyte solution
bet.	between
BET	benign epileptiform transients
BeV	billion electron volts
bf	bouillon filtrate (tuberculin)
B/F	balance forward (bookkeeping abbreviation); bound-free ratio; breast-feeding; brought forward
BF	black female; blastogenic factor; body fat; break-fast
BFC	benign febrile convulsion
BFGF	basic fibroblast growth factor
BFP	biologic false-positive (reaction)
BFR	blood flow rate; bone formation rate
BFT	bentonite flocculation test

BFU-E	burst-forming units — erythroid
BFVR	blood flow volume ratio
B-G	Bordet-Gengou (bacillus)
BG	blood glucose; bone graft; bucco-gingival
BGG	bovine gamma globulin
BGL	Bernard's granular layer
BGH	bovine growth hormone
B-glands	Bowman's glands
BGP	beta-glycero-phosphatase
BGSA	blood granulocyte specific activity
BGTT	borderline glucose tolerance test
BHA	butylated hydroxy-anisole
BHAPs	bis-hetero-aryl piperazines
B-HBA	beta-hydroxy-butyric acid
BHC	benzene hexa-chloride
b-HCG	beta-human chorionic gonadotrophin (hormone); pregnancy test (using blood sample)
B-HCG	beta-human chorionic gonadotrophin (hormone); pregnancy test (using blood sample)
BHD	BCNU, Hydroxyurea, DTIC
BHDV	BCNU, Hydroxyurea, DTIC, Vincristine
BHI	brain-heart infusion
BHK	baby hamster kidney
B-HS	beta-hemolytic streptococcus
BHT	butylated hydroxy-toluene
BH/VH	body hematocrit / venous hematocrit (ratio)
bi	biopsy; bisexual
Bi	Bismuth
BI	bacteriological index; base in; bowel impaction; brain injury; burn index
bib.	*bibe* (drink)
bicarb.	bicarbonate
b.i.d.	*bis in die* (twice a day)
BID	brought in dead
BIDS	brittle hair, impaired intelligence, decreased fertility, short stature
BIH	benign intracranial hypertension
BIHT	benign intracranial hyper-tension
bil.	bilateral
Bili	bilirubin
Bili-C	conjugated bilirubin
BIMA	bilateral internal mammary arteries
b.i.n.	*bis in nocte* (twice a night)

BIO	biological; biology
biol.	biological; biology
BiP	an immunoglobulin binding protein
bis	*bis* (twice)
bis in 7d.	*bis in septum diebus* (twice a week)
BIVAD	centrifugal left and right ventricular assist device
B&J	bone and joint
BJ	Bence Jones; biceps jerks
BJA	Bence Jones albumose
BJM	bones, joints, muscles
BJME	bone, joint, muscle examination
BJP	Bence Jones protein
bk.	book
Bk	Berkelium; book
BK	below knee; book
BKA	below knee amputation
BK-amp	below knee amputation
bkfst.	breakfast
BKV	BK virus
BKWP	below knee walking plaster
BL	base-line; black; bleeding; block; blood; blood loss; blue; bucco-labial; bucco-lingual; Burkitt's lymphoma
BLAD	border-line left axis deviation
BLB mask	Boothby-Lovelace-Bulbulian mask
BLB unit	Bessey-Lowry-Brock unit
bl. cult.	blood culture
bld.	blood
BLDG	building
BLE	both lower extremities
Bleo.	Bleomycin
Bleo-COMF	Bleomycin, CCNU, Oncovin, Methotrexate, Fluorouracil
BLG	beta-lacto-globulin
Blk	black; block
Blm.	Bleomycin
BLN	bronchial lymph nodes
BLOB	bladder obstruction
bl. pr.	blood pressure
BLS	basic life support
BLT	blood (clot) lysis time
BLU	Bessey-Lowry units
BLV	bovine leukemia virus
b.m.	*balneum maris* (sea-water bath)

BM	basal metabolism; black male; body mass; bone marrow; bone mass; bowel movement; bucco-mesial
BMA	British Medical Association
BMD	bone marrow depression
BME	bio-medical engineering; brief maximal effort
BMG	benign monoclonal gammopathy
B_2MG	beta-two-micro-globulin
BMI	body mass index
BMJ	British Medical Journal
BMK	birth-mark
BMOPP	Bleomycin, Methyldiamine, Oncovin, Procarbazine, Prednisone
BMP	Bleomycin, Methotrexate, Platinol; bone marrow pressure; bone morphogenic protein
BMR	basal metabolic rate
BMRTC	bone metastasizing renal tumor of childhood
BMS	Bachelor of Medical Science; burning mouth syndrome
BMT	bone marrow transplantation
BN	brachial neuritis
BNC	bladder neck contracture
BNLI	British National Lymphoma Investigation
BNMSE	Brief Neuropsychological Mental Status Examination
BNO	bladder neck obstruction
BNPA	bi-nasal pharyngeal airway
BNS	benign nephro-sclerosis
B&O	belladonna and opium
BO	bladder obstruction; body odor; bowel obstruction; bucco-occlusal
BOA	born on arrival; British Orthopaedic Association
BOAP	Bleomycin, Oncovin, Adriamycin, Prednisone
BOBA	beta-oxy-butyric acid
BOC	t-but-oxy-carbonyl
BOEA	ethyl biscoumacetate (Pelentan; Tromexan)
BOH	bundle of His
bol.	*bolus* (a large pill)
BOLD	Bleomycin, Oncovin, Lomustine, Dacarbazine
BOM	bilateral otitis media
BONP	Bleomycin, Oncovin, Natulan, Prednisolone
BOOP	bronchiolitis obliterans organizing pneumonia
BOP	BCNU, Oncovin, Prednisone
BOPP	Bleomycin, Oncovin, Procarbazine, Prednisone
b.p.	boiling point; base pair
B.P.	British Pharmacopeia (Pharmacopoeia)

BP	back-pressure; bed-pan; benzo-pyrene; birth-place; blood pressure; broncho-pleural; broncho-pulmonary; bucco-pulpal; by-pass
BPA	breast, pubic, axillary hair; British Paediatric Association
BPC	British Pharmaceutical Codex
BPD	bi-parietal diameter; broncho-pulmonary dysplasia
BPDLB	block in the posterioinferior division of the left branch
BPF	broncho-pulmonary fistula
B.Ph.	British Pharmacopeia (Pharmacopoeia)
BPH	benign prostatic hyperplasia; benign prostatic hypertrophy
BPHO	Business-Physician-Hospital Organization
BPHP	benign prostatic hyper-plasia
BPHT	benign prostatic hyper-trophy
Bpi	bytes per inch
BPIG	bacterial polysaccharide immune globulin
BPL	beta-propio-lactone
bpm	beats per minute
BPP	benzyl-penicillin potassium
BPRS	brief psychiatric rating scale
bps	beats per second
BPS	beats per second; benzyl-penicillin sodium; bilateral partial salpingectomy; breaths per second; bytes per second
BPSA	broncho-pulmonary segmental artery
BPV	bovine papilloma virus; benign positional vertigo
Bq	Becquerel (cell)
Br.	*Brucella*
Br	branch; brass; British; bright; Bromine; brother; brown
BR	bath-room; bed-rest; bed-room; bili-rubin; bladder re-construction; body reaction; brain; British; by report
brady.	bradycardia
brady/tachy	bradycardia / tachycardia (ratio)
BRAT	Baylor Rapid Autologous Transfusion
BRBC	bovine red blood cells
BRC	bladder re-construction
BrDU	bromo-deoxy-uridine
Brev.	sodium brevital
BRFS	behavior risk factor surveillance system
brk.	break
BRM	biological response modifier; biuret reactive material
Broncho.	bronchoscopy
BRP	bath-room privileges; bili-rubin production
BRTN-L	Burton's line

B.S.	Bachelor of Science; Bachelor of Surgery; *Baccalaureus Scientiae* (Bachelor of Science)
BS	before sleep; blood sugar; blood system; body system; bowel sounds; brain syndrome; breath sounds
BSA	bismuth-sulfite agar; bistrimethyl-silyl-acetamide; body surface area; bovine serum albumin
BSAEP	brain stem auditory evoked potential
BSAER	brain stem auditory evoked response
BSAP	brief short action potential
BSB	body surface burned
B.Sc.	*Baccalaureus Scientiae* (Bachelor of Science)
BSE	bilateral symmetrical and equal; breast self-examination
BSER	brain stem evoked response
BSF	B-lymphocyte stimulating factor
BSF-1	B-cell stimulatory factor 1
BSF-2	B-cell stimulatory factor 2
BSF-pl	B-cell stimulatory factor pl
B&S glands	Bartholin and Skene's glands
BSI	bound serum iron
BSL	bio-safety level; blood sugar level
BSN	Bachelor Science in Nursing; bowel sounds normal
BSO	bilateral salpingo-oophorectomy; buthionine sulf-oximine
BSOM	bilateral serious otitis media
BSP	brom-sul-phalein test; brom-sulfon-phthalein test
BS-par	Brown-Séquard's paralysis
BSR	basal skin resistance
BSS	balanced salt solution; black silk suture; buffered saline solution
BS-syn	Brown-Séquard's syndrome
BST	bismuth sodium triglycollamate; Bistrimate
BSTFA	bistrimethyl-silyl-tri-fluoro-acetamide
BSU	British Standard Units
BSUG	Bartholin, Skene, urethral glands
BT	balloon tamponade; bed-time; bladder tumor; bleeding time; brain tumor
BTB	break-through bleeding
BTE	behind the ear; behind the eye
BTL	bilateral tubal ligation
BTLS	basic trauma life support
BTMG	beta-2-micro-globulin
BTPS	body temperature and pressure, saturated with water vapor
BTS	Benedict's test for sugar

Btu	British Thermal Unit
BTU	British Thermal Unit
bu.	butyl
BU	Bodansky unit; burn unit
bull.	*bulliat* (let it boil)
BUN	blood urea nitrogen
BURD	5-bromodeoxy-uridine
BURK-L	Burkitt's lymphoma
but.	*butyrum* (butter)
BUT	break-up time; Butisol (butabarbital); Butyn (butacine)
BV	*balneum vaporis* (vapor bath); biological value; bi-ventricular blood vessel; blood volume
BVA	best (corrected) visual acuity
BVAD	bi-ventricular assist device
BVAP	BCNU, Vincristine, Adriamycin, Prednisone
BVAPP	BCNU, Velban, Cytoxan, Procarbazine, Prednisone
BVDS	Bleomycin, Velban, Doxorubicin, Streptozocin; Bleomycin, Vincristine, Doxorubicin, Streptozocin
BVCPP	BCNU, Velban, Cytoxan, Procarbazine, Prednisone
BVCPPB	BCNU, Velban, Cytoxan, Procarbazine, Prednisone, Bleomycin
BVH	bi-ventricular hypertrophy
BVI	blood vessel invasion
B virus.	herpes-virus simiae
BVM	broncho-vesicular markings
BVPP	BCNU, Oncovin, Procarbazine, Prednisone
BVR	Bureau of Vocational Rehabilitation
BVV	bovine vaginitis virus
BW	body water; body weight; boiling water; brain-washing; brain wave
BWD	bacillary white diarrhea (pullorum disease)
BWS	Beckwith-Wiedemann syndrome
bx	box
Bx	biopsy
bxs	boxes
bys.	bysma; byssinosis; byssocausis; byssus
bz	benzoyl
Bza	benzimidazole; benzymidazolyl
BzH	benzaldehyde
bzl	benzyl
BzOH	benzene-carboxylic acid

C

$\bar{c}$	*cum* (with)
©	confidential; copyright
c	calorie; *centum* (hundred); *cibus* (food); *circum* (around); *congius* (gallon); speed of light
C	calm; cancel; cancelled; candle; capacitance; capacitor; capacity; carbon; case; cathode; Caucasian; cell; Celsius; center; centigrade; centimeter; certified; certify; cervical; chest; Chlorambucil; Cisplatin; clear; clearance; clock; clone; clonus; Clostridium; closure; clubbing; cocaine; color; complement; complete; compliance; compound; contact; contraction; cough; coulomb; count; Cryptococcus; Curie; cyanosis; cycle; Cyclophosphamide; cylinder; cysteine; cytidine; cytosine; Cytoxan; kilo-calorie; vitamin C
C_s	caesarean section (cesarean section)
C_{II}	second cranial nerve
C^{14}	radio-active carbon
C_{alb}	albumin clearance
C_{am}	amylase clearance
C_{cr}	creatinine clearance
C_{in}	insulin clearance
C_{pah}	para-amino-hippurate clearance
C_T	correction factor for temperature
C_u	urea clearance
C1	first cervical vertebrae
C2	second cervical vertebrae
c/a	cash on account (bookkeeping abbreviation)
ca.	*circa* (about)
Ca	calcium; cancer; carcinoma
Ca^{++}	calcium ion
C&A	Clinitest and acetone
CA	cancer; carbonic anyhydrase; carcinoma; cardiac apnea; cardiac arrest; carotid artery; celiac artery; chronological age; cold agglutinin; common antigen; coronary artery; corpora amylacea; croup-associated; Cytoxan, Adriamycin

CAAT	computer-assisted axial tomography
CAB	coronary artery bypass
CABBS	California Bulletin Board System
CABG	coronary artery bypass graft
CABOP	Cytoxan, Adriamycin, Bleomycin, Oncovin, Prednisone
CABPS	coronary artery by-pass surgery
CABS	CCNU, Adriamycin, Bleomycin, Streptozotocin; coronary artery bypass surgery
CAC	cardio-acceleratory center
CACC	cathodal closure contraction
$CaCl_2$	calcium-chloride
CACMS	Committee on Accreditation of Canadian Medical Schools
$CaCO_3$	calcium-carbonate
CaC_2O_4	calcium-oxalate
CAD	computer-aided design; computer-assisted diagnosis; coronary artery disease; Cytoxan, Adriamycin, Dacarbazine
CAE	cellulose acetate electrophoresis
CAEV	caprine arthritis encephalitis virus
CAF	Cyclophosphamide, Adriamycin, Fluorouracil
CaF_2	calcium-fluoride
CAFA	carotid audio-frequency analysis
CAFP	California Academy of Family Physicians; Cytoxan, Adriamycin, Fluorouracil, Prednisone
CAFT	Cisplatin, Adriamycin, Fluorouracil, Teniposide; Clinitron air-fluidized therapy
CAFVP	Cytoxan, Adriamycin, Fluorouracil, Vincristine, Prednisone
CAG	chronic atrophic gastritis
CAH	chronic active hepatitis; congenital adrenal hyperplasia
CAHEA	Committee on Allied Health Education and Accreditation
CAHD	coronary atherosclerotic heart disease
CAHP	congenital adrenal hyperplasia
(Ca)i	calcium intercellular
CAI	computer-assisted instruction
C-AJCC	Clinical—American Joint Committee on Cancer
cal.	calender; caliber; calorie (small)
Cal.	calender; caliber; calorie (large)
calc.	calculate; calculation
CALD	chronic active liver disease

calef.	*calefac* (make warm); *calefactus* (warmed)
CALGB	cancer and acute leukemia group B
CALL	common acute lymphocytic leukemia
CALLA	common acute lymphoblastic leukemia antigen; common acute lymphocytic leukemia antigen
CALPAC	California Medical Political Action Committee
CAM	cell adhesion molecule; chorio-allantoic membrane; computer-aided manufacturing; contralateral axillary metastasis; Cytoxan, Adriamycin, Methotrexate
CAMB	Cyclophosphamide, Adriamycin, Methotrexate, Bleomycin
CAMEO	Cytoxan, Adriamycin, Methotrexate, Etoposide, Oncovin
CAMF	Cytoxan, Adriamycin, Methotrexate, Folinic acid
CAML	Cytoxan, Adriamycin, Methotrexate, Leucovorin
CAMLO	Cytosine, Arabinoside, Methotrexate, Leucovorin, Oncovin
camp.	campimeter; campimetry
cAMP	cyclic 3'5'-adenosine mono-phosphate
CAMP	Cytoxan, Adriamycin, Methotrexate, Procarbazine
CAMV	congenital anomaly of mitral valve
CaO	calcium-oxide
CAO	chronic airway obstruction; Cytoxan, Adriamycin, Oncovin
Ca(OH)$_2$	calcium-hydroxide
cap.	capacitor; *capiat* (let him take); capillus; *capsula* (capsule)
CAP	Capastat; capital; capsule; captain; cardiac action potential; catabolite (gene) activator protein; cellulose acetate phthalate; cystine amino-peptidase; Cytoxan, Adriamycin, Platinol; Cytoxan, Adriamycin, Prednisone
CAPBOP	Cytoxan, Adriamycin, Procarbazine, Bleomycin, Oncovin, Prednisone
CAPD	chronic ambulatory peritoneal dialysis; continuous ambulatory peritoneal dialysis
CAPH	California Association of Public Hospitals
CAPR	combined abdomino-perineal resection
CAR	Canadian Association of Radiologists
Carb.	carbohydrate
CARD	cardiac automatic resuscitative device
CARE	Center for AIDS Research and Education; Cooperative for American Relief to Everywhere
CAS	carotid artery stenosis; cartridge aspirating syringe; Chemical Abstracts Service

CASH	cruciform anterior spinal plate
CaSO$_4$	calcium-sulfate
CAST	Cardiac Arrhythmia Suppression Trial
cat.	catalog (catalogue); catalyst; *cataplasma* (a poultice)
CAT	California Association of Toxicologists; Children Apperception Test; chloramphenicol acetyl transferase; Chlormerodrin Accumulation Test; computer-assisted tomography; computerized axial tomography
cath.	*catharticus* (cathartic); catheter; catheterization; catheterize
cathd.	catheterized
CATH lab.	catheterization laboratory
CAT scan	computed axial tomography scan
CAT-SD	cat scratch disease
CATT scan	computed axial transverse tomography scan
CATV	community antenna television
Cauc.	Caucasian
CAUSE	California Association of Uniform Safety Employees
CAV	congenital absence of vagina; congenital adrenal virilism; Cyclophosphamide, Adriamycin, Vincristine
CAVB	complete atrio-ventricular block
CAVe	Cyclophosphamide, Adriamycin, Velban
CAVH	continuous arterio-venous hemofiltration
CAVHF	continuous arterio-venous hemo-filtration
CAVP	Cytoxan, Adriamycin, Vincristine, Prednisone
CAVUF	continuous arterio-venous ultra-filtration
CAWO	closing abductory wedge osteotomy
Cb	Columbium (Niobium)
C.B.	*Chirurgiae Baccalaureus* (Bachelor of Surgery)
CB	cervico-buccal; chocolate blood; chronic bronchitis
CB-3025	Melphalan
CBA	chronic bronchitis (with) asthma
CBBB	complete bundle branch block
CBC	complete bloodcell count
CBCC	complete blood-cell count
CBD	closed bladder drainage; common bile duct
CBE	Cytoxan, BCNU, Etoposide
CBF	cerebral blood flow; coronary blood flow
CBG	capillary blood gas; coronary bypass graft; corticosteroid-binding globulin; cortisol-binding globulin
CBP	Campylo-bacter pylori; chronic back pain
CBPP	contagious bovine pleuro-pneumonia

CBPS	chronic benign pain syndrome
CBR	complete bed rest
CBS	capillary blood sugar; chronic brain syndrome
CBV	CCNU, Bleomycin, Velban; central blood volume; cerebral blood volume; circulating blood volume; corrected blood volume
CBVD	CCNU, Bleomycin, Velban, Dexamethasone
CBVP	catheter balloon valvulo-plasty
CBW	chemical and biological warfare
cc	cubic centimeter (cubic centimetre)
CC	cardiac cycle; Caucasian child; cervical cyst; chief complaint; circulatory collapse; close call; close-captioned; closed-chain; closed-circuit; closing capacity; colony count; common cold; congenital cyst; contaminated culture; coraco-clavicular; cord compression; corpus callosum; costo-chondral; counter clockwise; creatinine clearance; critical care; critical case; critical condition; critical count
CCA	chick cell agglutination; chimpanzee coryza agent; circumflex coronary artery; common carotid artery; congenital contractual arachnodactyly
CCAT	conglutinating complement absorption test
CC&C	colony count and culture
CCC	cathodal closure clonus; cathodal closure contraction; chronic calculus cholecystitis
CCCl	cathodal closure clonus
CCCR	closed-chest cardiac resuscitation
CCDPHP	Center for Chronic Disease Prevention and Health Promotion
CCE	clubbing, cyanosis, edema
CCF	cephalin cholesterol flocculation; congestive cardiac failure; crystal-induced chemotactic factor
CCG	Children's Cancer Group
CCHD	cyanotic congenital heart disease
CCHS	congenital central hypoventilation syndrome
CCHVS	congenital central hypo-ventilation syndrome
CCI	chronic coronary insufficiency
CCK	chole-cysto-kinin
CCl_4	carbon tetra-chloride
CCM	critical care medicine; Cytoxan, CCNU, Methotrexate
CCMS	clean catch mid-stream
CCMSU	clean catch mid-stream urine

CCNU	cyclonexyl-chloroethyl-nitroso-urea (Lomustine)
CCP	cilio-cyto-phthoria
CCPR	cerebral cortex perfusion rate
CCRN	Critical Care Registered Nurse
CCS	California Children Services; Canadian Cardiovascular Society; Cronkhite-Canada Syndrome
CCSG	Children's Cancer Study Group
CCT	cathodal closure tetanus; computed cranial tomography
CCTG	computed cranial tomo-graphy
CCTV	closed-circuit television
CCU	coronary care unit; critical care unit; cardiac care unit
CCUP	colpo-cysto-urethro-pexy
CCV	CCNU, Cytoxan, Vincristine; conductivity cell volume
CCVPP	CCNU, Cytoxan, Velban, Procarbazine, Prednisone
CCW	counter clock-wise
c.d.	*conjugata diagonalis* (diagonal conjugate)
Cd	Cadmium
C&D	cystoscopy and dilatation
CD	cadaver donor; caesarean delivered; caesarean delivery; carbonate dehydratase; cardiac disease; cardiac dullness; Christmas disease; circular dischroism; cluster designation; color deficient; common duct; compact disc (disk); conduction defect; convulsive disorder; curative dose; cystic duct
CD_4	T-helper lymphocyte
CDA	cheno-deoxycholic acid; chloro-deoxy-adenosine; congenital dysery-thropietic anemia
CDAP	continuous distending airway pressure
C&DB	cough and deep breath
CDC	calculated date of confinement; California Department of Corrections; Center for Disease Control and Prevention
CDC-AIDS	Center for Disease Control for AIDS diagnosis
CDDP	cis-diamine-dichloro-platinum
CDGP	constitutional delay of growth and puberty
CDH	congenital diaphragm of hernia; congenital dislocation of hip; congenital dysplasia of hip
CDHS	California Department of Health Services
CDL	chloro-deoxy-lincomycin
cDNA	complementary deoxyribo-nucleic acid; copy DNA
CDP	continuous distending (airway) pressure; cytidine di-phosphate
CDR	computed digital radiography; cup disk ratio

CD-ROM	compact disc (disk) read-only memory
c.d.s.	cul-de-sac (French: a blind, pouch or sac, as the cecum)
Ce	Cerium
CE	California encephalitis; cardiac enlargement; chick embryo; Continuing Education
CEA	carcino-embryonic antigen; carotid end-arterectomy; cin-embryonic antigen; crystalline egg albumin
CEB	Carboplatin, Etoposide, Bleomycin
CEEV	Central European Encephalitis Virus
CEF	chick embryo fibroblast
CEJA	Council on Ethical and Judicial Affairs
CEM	CCNU, Etoposide, Methotrexate
CEN	Certified Emergency Nurse
CEO	chief executive officer
CEP	CCNU, Etoposide, Prednimustine; congenital erythropoietic porphyria
ceph.	cephalic
cer.	ceramide; certified; certify; ceruloplasmin
CER	conditioned emotional response; conditioned escape response
CES	central excitatory state
CESD	cholesteryl ester storage disease
CETP	cholesteryl ester transfer protein
CEU	Continuing Education Unit
CEV	Cyclophosphamide, Etoposide, Vincristine
CEVD	CCNU, Etoposide, Vindesine, Dexamethasone
cf.	*confer* (compare)
Cf	Californium
CF	cancer-free; carbol-fuchsin; cardiac failure; carried forward; centrifugal force; chest and face; Chiari-Frommel; Christmas factor; citrovorum factor; complement fixation; complement fixing; contractile force; count fingers; cystic fibrosis
CFA	complement-fixing antibody; complete Freund's adjuvant
c.f.f.	critical fusion frequency
CFIDS	chronic fatigue and immune dysfunction syndrome
cfm	cubic feet per minute
CFM	cerebral function monitor
CFMG	Commission on Foreign Medical Graduates
CFP	chronic false-positive; cystic fibrosis of the pancreas; Cytoxan, Fluorouracil, Prednisone
CFPT	Cytoxan, Fluorouracil, Prednisone, Tamoxifen

CFR	Code of Federal Regulations
cfs	cubic feet per second
CFS	chronic fatigue syndrome
CFT	complement fixation test
CFU	colony-forming unit
CFU-C	colony-forming unit — culture
CFU-E	colony-forming unit — erythroid
CFU-EOS	colony-forming unit — eosinophil
CFU-F	colony-forming unit — fibroblast
CFU-GEMM	colony-forming unit — granulocyte, erythrocyte, monocyte, megakaryocyte; colony-forming unit — granulocyte, erythrocyte, monocyte, megalokaryocyte
CFU-GM	colony-forming unit — granulocyte macrophage
CFU-L	colony-forming unit — lymphoid
CFU-M	colony-forming unit — megakarocyte
CFU-NM	colony-forming unit — neutrophil monocyte
CFU-S	colony-forming unit — spleen
CFWM	cancer-free white mouse
CG	Cardio-green (Indocyanine green = a diagnostic acid) chorionic gonadotropin; chronic glomerulonephritis; colloidal gold
CGb	chorionic gonadotropin — beta
CG-B	chorionic gonadotropin — beta
CGD	chronic granulomatous disease
c.gl.	correction (with) glasses
CGL	chronic granulocytic leukemia; correction (with) glasses
cgm	centi-gram
cGMP	cyclic 3'5'-guanyl mono-phosphate
CGN	chronic glomerulo-nephritis
CGNA	Canadian Gerontological Nursing Association
CG/OQ	cerebral glucose / oxygen quotient (ratio)
CGP	choline glycero-phosphatide; circulating granulocyte pool
CGS	cat-gut suture; centimeter-gram-second
CGT	chorionic gonado-tropin
CGTT	cortisol glucose tolerance test
ch.	chain; chaplain; chapter; chief; child; children; church
Ch[1]	Christ-church chromosome
CH	chest; cholesterol; chloral hydrate; Christian; crown-heel (length of fetus)
CH_4	marsh gas; methane
C_2H_2	acetylene

C_2H_4	ethylene
C_6H_6	benzene
CHA	congenital hypoplastic anemia; cyclo-hexyl-amine
CHAC	Cytoxan, Hexamethylmelamine, Adriamycin, Carboplatin
CHAD	Cytoxan, Hexamethylmelamine, Adriamycin, DDP
CHAMOA	Cytoxan, Hydroxyurea, Actinomycin D, Methotrexate, Oncovin, Adriamycin
CHAMPUS	Civilian Health and Medical Program of the Uniformed Services
CHAP	Cytoxan, Hexamethylmelamine, Adriamycin, Platinol
chart.	*charta* (paper)
Ch.B.	*Chirurgiae Baccalaureus* (Bachelor of Surgery)
CHB	complete heart block
Ch.D.	*Chirurgiae Doctor* (Doctor of Surgery)
CHD	child-hood disease; child; children; chronic heart disease; congenital heart disease; congenital hip dysplasia; congestive heart disease; coronary heart disease
CHDP	Child Health and Disability Prevention
CHDTP	Child Health and Disability Treatment Program
ChE	cholin-esterase
chem.	chemical; chemistry; chemo-therapy
CHF	congestive heart failure
CHFP	Cytoxan, Hexamethylmelamine, Fluorouracil, Platinol
CHH	cartilage-hair hypoplasia
CHI	closed-head injury
ChINA	chronic infectious neuropathic agent; chronic infectious neurotropic agent
CHL	Chlorambucil; Chloramphenicol; crown-heel length
CHLOR-M	chlorpheniramine maleate (anti-histamine)
ChlVPP	Chlorambucil, Vinblastine, Procarbazine, Prednisone
Ch.M	*Chirurgiae Magister* (Master of Surgery)
CHMD	clinical hyaline membrane disease
CHN	central hemorrhagic disease
CHO	Chinese hamster ovary; Cytoxan, Hydroxydaunomycin, Oncovin
CHOB	Cytoxan, Hydroxydaunomycin, Oncovin, Bleomycin
chol.	cholesterol
CHOO	chronic hepatic outflow obstruction
CHOP	Cytoxan, Hydroxydaunomycin, Oncovin, Prednisone
CHOPB	Cytoxan, Hydroxydaunomycin, Oncovin, Prednisone, Bleomycin

CHO-XRT	Cytoxan, Hydroxydaunomycin, Oncovin — radiation therapy
CHP	chloral hydrate poisoning; Community Health Plan
CHPA	Community Health Purchasing Alliance
CHPAs	Community Health Purchasing Alliances
CHPX	chicken-pox
Chr.	Christian; chronic
CHR	Christian; chronic hypercapnic respiratory (failure)
CHRF	chronic hypercapnic respiratory failure
CHS	contact hyper-sensitivity; Chediak-Higashi syndrome
Ci	Curie
CI	cardiac index; cardiac insufficiency; cephalic index; cerebral infarction; chemotherapeutic index; colloidal iron; color index; confidence interval; coronary insuf-ficiency; crystalline insulin
CIA	CCNU, Isophosphamide, Adriamycin
cib.	*cibus* (food)
CIC	cardio-inhibitory center; carpal instability complex; circulating immune complexes
CICF	crystal-induced chemotactic factor
CICU	cardiac intensive care unit ; coronary intensive care unit
CID	carpal instability dissociative; cytomegalic inclusion disease
CIDP	chronic inflammatory demyelinating polyradiculoneuropathy
CIDS	cellular immuno-deficiency syndrome
CIEP	counter immuno-electro-phoresis
CIF	Claims Inquiry Form; clone-inhibiting factor
CIG	cigarette; cigarettes; cytoplasmic immuno-globulin
CIN	cervical intraepithelial neoplasia; chronic interstitial nephritis
CIND	carpal instability non-dissociative
cir.	circle; circular; circumcision
circ.	circle; circular; circumcision
circum.	circumcision; circumference
CIS	Cancer Information Service; carcinoma in-situ; central inhibitory state; Cisplatin (Platinol)
c.i.s.a.	*coque in sufficiente aqua* (boil in sufficient water)
CISCA	Cisplatin, Cyclophosphamide, Adriamycin
cito disp.	*cito dispensetur* (let it be dispensed quickly)
CIVD	cold-induced vaso-dilation
CIXU	constant infusion excretory urogram
CIXUG	constant infusion excretory uro-gram

CJD	Creutzfeld-Jakob disease
CK	check; creatine kinase
cl	centi-liter (centi-litre) clear; clearance; close; cloudy; corpus luteum
Cl	cervico-lingual; chloride; chlorine; class; Clostridium
Cl⁻	chloride ion
CL_{ss}	total systematic clearance
CLAS	cholesterol-lowering atherosclerosis study; congenital localized absence of skin
CLBBB	complete left bundle branch block
CL&CP	cleft lip and cleft palate
CLD	chronic liver disease; chronic lung disease; cleared
CLH	chronic lobular hepatitis
CLIA	Clinical Laboratory Improvement Amendments
CLILP	corticotropin-like intermediate lobe peptide
CLIP	corticotropin-like intermediate (lobe) peptide
CLL	chronic lymphatic leukemia; chronic lymphoblastic leukemia; chronic lymphocytic leukemia
CLLE	columnar-lined lower esophagus
CLMA	Clinical Laboratory Management Association
CLO	cod liver oil
CLPN	Cancer Liaison Physician Network
CLS	chronic lymphadenopathy syndrome
CLSH	corpus luteum-stimulating hormone
CLSL	chronic lympho-sarcoma leukemia
CLT	Clinical Laboratory Technologist; clot-lysis time
c.m.	*cras mane* (tomorrow morning)
cm	centi-meter (centi-metre)
cm²	square centimeter (square centimetre)
cm³	cubic centimeter (cubic centimetre)
cM	centi-Morgan
Cm	Curium
CM	capreo-mycin; cardiac monitor; cow's milk; chloroquine-mepacrine; clinical management; clinical modification; cochlear micro-phonics; costal margin
CMA	California Medical Association; Canadian Medical Association; Certified Medical Assistant
CMAJ	*Canadian Medical Association Journal*
CMC	carpo-meta-carpal; carboxy-methyl-cellulose; critical micelle concentration; Cytoxan, Methotrexate, CCNU
CMD	cerebro-macular degeneration; Current Medical Dialog (Dialogue)

CME	Continuing Medical Education; Council on Medical Education; cystoid macular edema
CMF	chondro-myxoid fibroma; Cyclophosphamide, Methotrexate, Fluorouracil
CMFP	Cytoxan, Methotrexate, Fluorouracil, Prednisone
CMFT	Cyclophosphamide, Methotrexate, Fluorouracil, Tamoxifen
CMFVP	Cytoxan, Methotrexate, Fluorouracil, Vincristine, Prednisone
CMG	cysto-metro-gram
CMGN	chronic membranous glomerulo-nephritis
CMI	cell-mediated immunity; cyto-megalic inclusion
CMID	cyto-megalic inclusion disease
c/min	cycles per minute
CMJ	carpo-metacarpal joint
CML	cell-mediated lymphocytotoxicity; cell-mediated lympholysis; chronic myelocytic leukemia; chronic myelogenous leukemia
cmm	cubic milli-meter (cubic milli-metre)
CMM	cutaneous malignant melanoma
CMML	chronic myelo-monocytic leukemia
CMN	cystic medial necrosis
CMN-AA	cystic medial necrosis of the ascending aorta
CMO	cardiac minute output
CMoL	chronic monoblastic leukemia; chronic monocytic leukemia
CMOPP	Cytoxan, Methydiamine, Oncovin, Procarbazine, Prednisone
CMOS	complementary metal oxide semiconductor
CMP	capillary membrane pressure; cardio-myo-pathy; CCNU, Procarbazine, Methotrexate; cytidine mono-phosphate
CMR	cerebral metabolic rate; crude mortality rate
CMRG	cerebral metabolic rate of glucose
CMRNG	chromosomally mediated resistant *Neisseria gonorrhoeae*
CMRO$_2$	cerebral metabolic rate of oxygen
CMRR	common mode rejection rate
c.m.s.	*cras mane sumendus* (to be taken tomorrow morning)
CMS	circulation muscle sensation
CMSP	County Medical Services Program
CMT	Certified Medical Transcriptionist; circus movement tachycardia; combined modality therapy
CMT-disease	Charcot-Marie-Tooth disease (peroneal muscular atrophy)

cmte.	committee
CMU	chlorophenyl-dimethyl-urea; monuron
CMV	Cisplatin, Methotrexate, Vinblastine; continuous mandatory ventilation; cyto-megalo-virus
c.n.	*cras nocte* (tomorrow night)
CN	cranial nerve; cya-nide; cya-nogen
CNA	California Nurses' Association
CNE	chronic nervous exhaustion
CNHD	congenital nonspherocytic hemolytic disease
CNL	cardiolipin natural lecithin
CNM	Certified Nurse Midwife
CNP	continuous negative pressure
c.n.s.	*cras nocte sumendus* (to be taken tomorrow night)
CNS	central nervous system; culture and sensitivity
CNV	conative negative variation; contingent negative variation
c/o	care of; check out
Co	Cobalt
CO	carbon monoxide; cardiac output; castor oil; centric occlusion; Certified Orthotist; complaints of; corneal opacity
CO_2	carbon dioxide
CoA	coenzyme A
COA	Canadian Orthopaedic Association
COAD	chronic obstructive airway disease
coag.	coagulate; coagulation
COAP	Cytoxan, Oncovin, Ara-C, Prednisone
COAPB	Cytoxan, Oncovin, Ara-C, Prednisone, Bleomycin
COATS	Comprehensive Occupational Assessment and Training System
COBMAM	Cytoxan, Oncovin, Bleomycin, Methotrexate, Adriamycin, MeCCNU
COBRA	Consolidated Omnibus Budget Reconciliation Act
COBS	caesarean-obtained barrier-sustained
COBT	chronic obstruction of biliary tract
COC	calcifying odontogenic cyst; cathodal opening clonus; cathodal opening contraction
cochl.	*cochleare* (a spoonful)
cochl. amp.	*cochleare amplum* (a heaping spoonful)
cochl. mag.	*cochleare magnum* (a tablespoonful)
cochl. med.	*cochleare medium* (a dessert spoonful)
cochl. par.	*cochleare parvum* (a teaspoonful)
COCl	cathodal opening clonus
coct.	*coctio* (boiling)

cod.	codeine
COD	cause of death
coef.	coefficient
COEPS	cortically originating extra pyramidal system
COGME	Council on Graduate Medical Education
COGTT	cortisone-primed oral glucose tolerance test
COH	carbohydrate
CoHb	carboxy-hemoglobin
col.	*cola* (strain); collect; collected; collection; college; collegiate; column
colat.	*colatus* (strained)
COLD	chronic obstructive lung disease
colet.	*coletur* (let it be strained)
collut.	*collutorium* (mouthwash)
collyr.	*collyrium* (an eyewash)
color.	*coloretur* (let it be colored)
COLTA	Colwell-Tamplin
com.	*commisce* (mix together)
COM	Cytoxan, Oncovin, Methotrexate
COMAA	Cytoxan, Oncovin, Methotrexate, Adriamycin, Ara-C
COMB	Cytoxan, Oncovin, Methotrexate, Bleomycin
COMF	Cytoxan, Oncovin, Methotrexate, Fluorouracil
COMLA	Cytoxan, Oncovin, Methotrexate, Leucovorin, Ara-C
COMLEC	Cytoxan, Oncovin, Methotrexate, Leucovorin, Etoposide, Cytarabine
comp.	complete; complicating; complication; composite; composition; *compositus* (compound); comprehensive
COMP	Cyclophosphamide, Oncovin, Methotrexate, Prednisone
COMS	Collaborative Ocular Melanoma Study
COMT	catechol-o-methyl transferase
conc.	concentrated; concentration; concise
concis.	*concisus* (cut)
CONF	conference; confirmation
config.	configuration; configure
cong.	congenital; congestion; *congius* (gallon); congress
cons.	*conserva* (keep); constant; consult; consultation
cons	consult; consultation
cont.	*continuetur* (continue; let it be continued); *contusus* (bruised)
contd.	continued
contr.	contraction; contrary
cont. rem.	*cintinuetur remedia* (let the medicines be continued)

cop.	copper; *copulatio* (copulation; sexual intercourse); copy
COP	colloidal oncotic pressure; colloidal osmotic pressure; copodyskinesia; copremesis; coprolagnia; coprolalia; coprolith; coprology; coprophagy; coprophilia; coproporphyrin; coproza; copula; Cyclophosphamide, Oncovin, Prednisone
COPA	Cytoxan, Oncovin, Prednisone, Adriamycin
COPAB	Cytoxan, Oncovin, Prednisone, Adriamycin, Bleomycin
COPAL	Cytoxan, Oncovin, Prednisone, Adriamycin, Lomustine
COPB	Cytoxan, Oncovin, Prednisone, Bleomycin
COPBAM	Cytoxan, Oncovin, Prednisone, Bleomycin, Adriamycin, Matulane
COPC	cerebral and overall performance categories; community-oriented primary care
COPD	chronic obstructive pulmonary disease
COPE	chronic obstructive pulmonary emphysema
COPP	CCNU, Oncovin, Procarbazine, Prednisone; Cytoxan, Oncovin, Procarbazine, Prednisone
coq.	*coque* (boil)
CoQ	coenzyme Q
coq. in s.a.	*coque in sufficiente aqua* (boil in sufficient water)
coq. s.a.	*coque secundum artem* (boil properly)
cor.	coordinate; corner; coroner; correct; corrected; correspond; correspondence; corresponding
CORA	conditioned orientation reflex audiometry
CORD	chronic obstructive respiratory disease
CORF	comprehensive outpatient rehabilitation facility
cort.	*cortex* (bark)
COS	Canadian Ophthalmological Society; cosine
cot.	*cotula* (a measure)
COT	cathodal opening tetanus
COTA	Certified Occupational Therapy Assistance
COTH	Council of Teaching Hospitals
cp	centi-poise (CGS unit of viscosity); *comparare* (compare)
cP	centi-poise (CGS unit of viscosity)
C&P	cystoscopy and pyelography
C/P	cholestrol / phospholipid (ratio)
CP	candle power; capillary pressure; carotid pressure; cerebral palsy; Certified Prosthetist; chemically pure; chest pain; chloro-purine; chloroquine primaquine; chronic pyelonephritis; cleft palate; closing pressure; copro-porphyrin; cor pulmonale; creatine phosphokinase; Cyclophosphamide, Prednisone

CPA	cardio-pulmonary arrest; carotid phon-angiography; cerebellar pontine angle; cerebello-pontine angle; chloro-phenyl-alanine; costo-phrenic angle; cyclo-phosph-amide
CPAN	Certified Post Anesthesia Nurse
CPAP	continuous positive airway pressure
CPAT	cerebello-pontine angle tumor
CPATS	cerebello-pontine angle tumor syndrome
CPB	cardio-pulmonary bypass; competitive protein binding; Cytoxan, Platinol, BCNU
CPBA	competitive protein-binding assay
CPC	central posterior curve; cetyl-pyridinium chloride; chronic passive congestion; clinico-pathological conference
CPCR	cardio-pulmonary cerebral resuscitation
CPCRA	Community Programs for Clinical Research on AIDS
cpd.	compound
CPD	cephalo-pelvic disproportion; citrate-phosphate-dextrose; continuous peritoneal dialysis
CPDA	citrate-phosphate-dextrose adenine
CPDD	calcium pyrophosphate deposition disease; cis-platinum-diamine-dichloride
CPE	chronic pulmonary emphysema; clubbing and pitting edema; cyto-pathic effect
CPEO	chronic progressive external ophthalmoplegia
CPG	capillary blood gas
CPH	chronic persistent hepatitis
CPI	coronary prognostic index
CPIP	chronic pulmonary insufficiency of prematurity
CPK	creatine phospho-kinase
cpl.	complete
c.p.m.	cycles per minute; counts per minute
CPM	CCNU, Procarbazine, Methotrexate; central pontine myelinolysis; continuous passive motion
CPN	chronic pyelo-nephritis
CPNA	Certified Pediatric Nurses' Association
CPNP	Certified Pediatric Nurse Practitioner
CPOB	Cytoxan, Prednisone, Oncovin, Bleomycin
CPP	capillary perfusion pressure; cerebral perfusion pressure
CPPB	continuous positive pressure breathing
CPPD	calcium pyro-phosphate dihydrate (disease)
CPPV	continuous positive pressure ventilation
CPR	cardio-pulmonary resuscitation; crystal production rate
c.p.s.	cycles per second (Hertz)

CPS	carbamoyl phosphate synthetase; cardio-pulmonary support; Center for Preventive Services; characters per second
CPSOP	Comprehensive Perinatal Services Outreach Program
CPT	chest physio-therapy; current procedural terminology
CPU	central processing unit
CPX	complete physical examination
CPZ	chlor-proma-zine
CQ	chloroquine-quinine; circadian quotient
c.r.	*continuetur remedium* (let the medicine be continued)
Cr	chrome; Chromium; cream; creatinine; credit (book-keeping abbreviation)
CR	cardio-respiratory; cathode ray; class rate; cold recombinant; colon resection; complement receptor; complete remission; complete response; conditioned reflex; conditioned response; creatinine; critical reaction; crown-rump
CR_1	first cranial nerve
CRA	central retinal artery
cranio.	craniopharyngioma
CRAO	central retinal artery occlusion
crast.	*crastinus* (for tomorrow)
CRBBB	complete right bundle branch block
CRBP	cellular retinol binding protein
CRC	colo-rectal cancer
CrCl	creatinine clearance
CRCS	Canadian Red Cross Society
CRD	chronic renal disease; chronic respiratory disease
CRE	cumulative radiation effect
creat.	creatinine
CReG	cross-reactive group (of HLA antigens)
CREN	constant rate enteral nutrition
CREST	Calcinosis cutis, Raynaud's phenomenon, Esophageal dysmotility, Scleroderma, Telangiectasia
CRF	chronic renal failure; chronic respiratory failure; closed reduction fixation; corticotropin-releasing factor
CRG	chest roentgeno-gram
CRGHA	cross-reactive group of HLA antigens
CRH	corticotropin-releasing hormone
CRIS	controlled-release infusion system
crit.	critical; hematocrit
CRITOE	Capitellum, Radial head, Internal condyle, Trochlea, Olecranon, External condyle

CRL	crown-rump length
CRM	Certified Reference Materials; cross-reacting material
cRNA	chromosomal ribo-nucleic acid
CRNA	Certified Registered Nurse Anesthetist
CRO	cathode-ray oscillograph; cathode-ray oscilloscope
CROG	cathode-ray oscillo-graph
CROP	Cytoxan, Rubidazone, Oncovin, Prednisone
CROS	cathode-ray oscillo-scope
CRP	C-reactive protein
CRS	Chinese Restaurant Syndrome; colon-rectal surgery
CR/SR	coccyx resection / sacral resection
CRST	Calcinosis cutis, Raynaud's phenomenon, Sclerodactyl, Telangiectasia
CRT	cathode-ray tube; Certified Respiratory Therapist; copper reduction test; corrected ray tube; court
CRTT	Certified Respiratory Therapy Technician
CRU	Clinical Research Unit
CRV	central retinal vein
CRVO	central retinal vein occlusion
CRVS	California Relative Value Studies
crypt.	cryptomenorrhea; cryptomenorrhoea; cryptomnesia
crys.	crystal; crystalline, crystallization
cryst.	crystal; crystalline, crystallization
c/s	caesarean section; cycles per second (Hertz)
Cs	Cesium
C&S	culture and sensitivity; conjuctiva and sclera
CS	caesarean section; cardiovascular system; cash on account (bookkeeping abbreviation); chondroitin sulfate; Clinical Specialist; clinical stage; cockup splint; cold sore; conditioned stimulus; coronary sinus; corpus striatum; cyclo-serine
c.s.a.	*coque secundum artem* (boil properly)
CSA	canavanino-succinic acid; chondroitin sulfate A; colon-stimulating activity; compressed spectral assay
CSAA	Child Study Association of America
CSB	conserved sequence block
c.s.c.	coup sur coup (French: in small doses at short intervals)
C-section	caesarean section; cesarean section
CSF	cerebro-spinal fluid; colony-stimulating factor
CSGBI	Cardiac Society of Great Britain and Ireland
CSH	carotid sinus hypersensitivity; chronic subdural hematoma; cortical stromal hyperplasia
CsI	Cesium iodide

CSM	cerebral spinal meningitis; chorionic somato-mammotropin
CSMI	cardiogenic shock (following acute) myocardial infarction
CSN	carotid sinus nerve
CSNRT	corrected sinus node recovery time
CSOM	chronic suppurative otitis media
CSP	Christian Science Practitioner
C-spine	cervical spine (films)
CSR	Cheyne-Stokes respiration; cortisol secretion rate; corrected sedimentation rate
CSS	carotid sinus stimulation
cST	centi-stoke
CST	Central Standard Time; contraction stress test; convulsive shock therapy
csTNM	clinical surgical tumor, node, metastasis (evaluation)
CSU	catheter specimen of urine
CT	calci-tonin; cardio-thoracic; carotid tracing; carpal tunnel; cerebral thrombosis; cervical traction; chemotherapy; chlorothiazide; circulation time; clotting time; coagulation time; collecting time; collecting tubule; collection time; computed tomography; computerized tomography; connective tissue; contraction time; Coomb's test; corneal transplant; coronary thrombosis; corrected transposition; corrective therapy; counselling and testing; count; court; crest time; critical time; Cyto-Technologist
CTA	Canadian Tuberculosis Association; chromo-tropic acid; clear to auscultation
CTAB	cetyl-trimethyl-ammonium bromide (cetrimonium bromide)
CTAT	computed trans-axial tomography; computerized transverse axial tomography
CTC	chlor-tetra-cycline (Biomycin)
CTCA	California Tuberculosis Controllers Association
CTCL	cutaneous T-cell lymphoma
$ctCO_2$	concentration of total carbon dioxide
CTD	carpal tunnel decompression; chest tube drainage; congenital thymic dysplasia
CTEP	Cancer Therapy Evaluation Program
CTG	computed tomo-graphy; computerized tomo-graphy
CTH	ceramide tri-hexoside
CTL	cytotoxic T-lymphocyte

CTLP	cytotoxic T-lymphocyte precursor
CTM-EEG	computed tomographic mapping of electro-encephalo-gram
CTP	cytidine tri-phosphate
CTR	cardio-thoracic ratio; carpal tunnel release; center; counter
CTRL	control
CTS	carpal tunnel syndrome; computed tomography scan
CTT	computed transaxial tomography
CTX	Cytoxan
CTX-DOX	Cytoxan, Doxorubicin
CTX-P	Cytoxan, Platinol
CTZ	chemoreceptor trigger zone; Chloro-thia-zide
Cu	cubic; *Cuprum* (copper)
CU	close-up
CUC	chronic ulcerative colitis
cuj.	*cujus* (of which)
cuj. lib.	*cujus libet* (of any you wish)
culdos.	culdoscope; culdoscopy
cum.	cumulative
CuO	cupric-oxide
CUSA	Cavitron Ultrasonic Surgical Aspirator
CUU	cross (end-to-end) uretero-ureterostomy
c.v.	*cras vespere* (tomorrow evening); *curriculum vitae* (course of life; résumé)
CV	cardio-vascular; cell volume; central venous; cerebro-vascular; closing volume; color vision; cresyl violet
CVA	cardio-vascular accident; cerebro-vascular accident; costo-vertebral angle; Cytoxan, Vincristine, Adriamycin
CVAT	costo-vertebral angle tenderness
CVB	CCNU, Vinblastine, Bleomycin; chorionic villus biopsy
CVC	central venous catheter
CVD	cardio-vascular disease; cerebro-vascular disease; collagen vascular disease; color vision deviant
CVF	Cytoxan, Vincristine, Fluorouracil
CVH	combined ventricular hypertrophy
CVHG	common variable hypogamma-globulinemia
CVI	common variable immunodeficiency
CVID	common variable immuno-deficiency
C-virus	Coxsackie virus
CVM	Cytoxan, Vincristine, Methotrexate

c.v.o.	*conjugata vera obstetrica* (obstetric conjugate diameter of pelvic inlet)
CVOD	cerebro-vascular obstructive disease
CVP	central venous pressure; Cytoxan, Vincristine, Prednisone
CVPP	CCNU, Velban, Procarbazine, Prednisone; Cyclophosphamide, Velban, Procarbazine, Prednisone
CVR	cardio-vascular renal; cerebro-vascular resistance
CVRD	cardio-vascular renal disease
CVRI	cardio-vascular resistance index
CVS	cardio-vascular surgery; cardio-vascular system; chorionic villus sampling; clean voided specimen
CVT	costo-vertebral tenderness
c/w	compare with; consistent with
CW	chemical warfare; chest wall; clean water; clock-wise; cold water
C-wave	continuous wave
CWDBF	cell wall deficient bacterial forms
CWI	cardiac work index
CWP	coal-worker's pneumoconiosis
Cx	cervix; convex; cylindrical lens axis
CXR	chest X-Ray
Cy	Cytoxan; cyanogen
CY	calender year
CyAD	Cytoxan, Adriamycin, Dacarbazine
cyath.	*cyathus* (glassful)
cyath. vin.	*cyathus vinosus* (glassful of wine)
Cyc	cycle; Cyclophosphamide
cyclic AMP	cyclic adenosine mono-phosphate
cyclic GMP	cyclic guanosine mono-phosphate
CYE	charcoal yeast extract
cyl.	cylinder; clyndrical
cyl. lens	cylindrical lens
cys.	cysteine; cystine
CYSTO	cystoscopy; cystogram
CyVADIC	Cytoxan, Vincristine, Adriamycin, Dimethyl-Imidazole-Carboxamide
CyVMAD	Cytoxan, Vincristine, Methotrexate, Dacarbazine
CZ	Central Zone
CZI	Crystalline Zinc Insulin

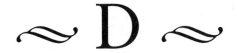

D

ΔALA	delta-amino-levulinic acid
/d	per day
d.	*da* (give); delta; *detur* (let it be given); *dexter* (right); *diem* (24 hours); *dies* (day); *dosis* (dose)
D	dark; date; daughter; Daunorubicin; day; dead; death; degree; delete; delta; density; derivative; Deuterium; Deuteron; Dexamethasone; dextro; dextrose; diagnosis; diameter; died; diet; dimension; diopter; director; distal; distance; diurnal; dog; dorsal; dose; *dosis* (dose); drowsy; duration; dwarf; vitamin D
D_5	dextrose 5% in water
D_M	diffusing capacity of the alveolar-capillary membrane
D_{max}	dose maximum (maximum dose)
2D	2-dimension
3D	3-dimension
D/A	date of accident; date of action; date of arrival; did not apply; Digital-to-Analog conversion; Digital-to-Analog converter; discharge with advice; do not apply
DA	degenerative arthritis; delayed action; deoxy-adenosine; developmental age; Dietetic Assistant; Digital-to-Analog (conversion); Digital-to-Analog (converter); direct access; direct agglutination; dis-aggregated; Dop-amine (3,4-dihydroxyphenethylamine); ductus arteriosus
DAB	4-dimethyl-aminoazo-benzene
DAC	Digital-to-Analog conversion; Digital-to-Analog converter
DACT	Dactinomycin
DADDS	di-acetyl-diamino-diphenyl-sulfone
DADP	deoxy-adenosine-di-phosphate
DAEC	diffuse adhering *Escherichia coli*
DAF	decay-activating factor; decay-accelerating factor
DAG	di-acyl-glycerol; disto-axio-gingival
DAGT	direct anti-globulin test
DAH	disordered action of heart
DAI	disto-axio-incisal

D-ALA	delta-amino-levulinic acid
DAM	di-acetyl-monoxime
DAMP	deoxy-adenosine mono-phosphate
DAO	di-amine oxidase
DAP	Dapsone; dihydroxy-acetone phosphate
DAPT	Daptazole; direct agglutination pregnancy test
d.a.s.f.	*donec alvus soluta fuerit* (until bowels are opened)
DAT	Daunomycin, Ara-C, Thioguanine; diet as tolerated; differential agglutination test; Digital Audio Tape; diphtheria anti-toxin; direct agglutination test; direct anti-globulin test
DATP	deoxy-adenosine tri-phosphate
DAV	Dacarbazine, Doxorubicin, Vincristine
db.	deci-bel
DB	Dextran blue; disto-buccal
DBA	di-benz-anthracene
DBCL	dilute blood clot lysis (method)
DBCP	di-bromo-chloro-propane
DBH	diameter at breast height
DBI	development-at-birth index
dbl.	double
DBP	diastolic blood pressure; disto-bucco-pulpal
DBS	Denis Browne Splint; despeciated bovine serum; diminished breath sounds
D&C	dilatation and curettage
D/C	direct count; discharge; discontinue; discontinued
D.C.	direct (electrical) current; Doctor of Chiropractic
DC	day care; dendritic cells; Dental Corps; deoxy-cholate; deoxy-cytidine; *dens caninus*; diarrhea, constipation; diphenylarsine cyanide; discharge; dis-continue; dis-continued; disto-cervical; double concave
DCA	deoxycholate-citrate agar; Department of Consumer Affairs; desoxy-corticosterone acetate
DCC	Digital Compact Cassette
DCCE	Department of Cancer Control and Epidemiology
DCCT	Diabetic Control and Complications Trials
DCDP	deoxy-cytidine di-phosphate
DCF	direct centrifugal flotation
DCFM	Doppler Color Flow Mapping
DCG	disodium cromo-glycate
D.C.H.	Diploma in Child Health
DCH	delayed cutaneous hypersensitivity
DCHFB	di-chloro-hexa-fluoro-butane

DCHS	delayed cutaneous hyper-sensitivity
DCI	di-chloro-isoproterenol
DCIS	ductal carcinoma in-situ
DCLS	deoxycholate-citrate-lactose-saccharose
DCM	di-chloro-methotrexate; dilated cardio-myopathy
DCMP	Daunorubicin, Cyclocytidine, Mercaptopurine, Prednisone; deoxy-cytidine-mono-phosphate
$D_L CO$	Carbon monoxide diffusing capacity of the lung
DCOG	Diploma of the College of Obstetricians and Gynaecologists
$D_L CO$-SB	Carbon monoxide diffusing capacity—single breath
DCP	dibasic-calcium-phosphate
DCS	dorsal column stimulator
DCT	deep chest therapy; direct Coombs' test
DCTMA	desoxy-corticosterone-tri-methyl-acetate
DCTP	deoxy-cytidine-tri-phosphate
DCTPA	desoxy-corticosterone-tri-phenyl-acetate
DCV	Dacarbazine, CCNU, Vincristine
DCx	double convex
d/d	dated; delivered
d.d.	*detur ad* (let it be given to)
dd	dated; delivered
DD	delivery date differential diagnosis; discharge diagnosis; dry dressing; due date
DDAVP	1-desamino-8-d-arginine vasopressin (Desmopressin)
DDC	di-deoxy-cytidine; diethyl-dithio-carbamate
DDD	degenerative disc disease; dense deposit disease; dichloro-diphenyl-dichloroethane
DDDE	dichloro-diphenyl-dichloro-ethylene
DDH	dissociated double hypertropia
DDI	di-deoxy-inosine
d.d.i.d.	*de die in diem* (from day to day)
DDMP	diamino-dichlorophenyl-methyl-pyrimidine
DDP	diamine-dichloro-platinum (Cisplatin; Platinol)
D.D.S.	Doctor of Dental Surgery
DDS	4,4-diamino-diphenyl-sulfone (Dapsone); dystrophy-dystocia syndrome
D.D.Sc.	Doctor of Dental Science
DDT	dichloro-diphenyl-trichloroethane (Dicophane)
DDTC	diethyl-di-thio-carbamate
DDVP	dimethyl-dichloro-vinyl phosphate (Dichlorvos)
DDx	differential diagnosis
De.	December

D&E	dilatation and evacuation; dilation and extraction (abortion)
DEAE	di-ethyl-amino-ethanol
DEBA	di-ethyl-barbituric acid
deb. spis.	*debita spissitudine* (of proper consistency)
dec.	*decanta* (pour off); decrement
Dec.	decant; deceased; December; decrease
DEC	deceased; December; dendritic epidermal cell
decomp.	decompensation; decompose; decomposition; decompound; decompress; decompression
decr.	decrement; decrease
decub.	*decubitus* (lying down)
DED	diabetic eye disease
DEEG	depth electro-encephalo-gram
def	charge deferred (bookkeeping abbreviation)
def.	*defaecatio* (defecation); defer; defile; defrost
DEF	decayed, extracted, filled; defaction; deficiency
defib.	defibrillate; defibrillation
DEG	degeneration; degree; depth electro-graphy
deglut.	*deglutiatur* (let it be swallowed)
del.	delivery (obstetric)
Dem.	Demerol
DEMO	demonstration
dep.	*depuratus* (purified)
DEPT	department; departure
derm.	*dermis* (skin); dermatology
DERV	duck embryo rabies vaccine
d.e.s.	*detur et signetur* (let it be given and labelled)
DES	di-ethyl-stilbestrol; diffuse esophageal spasm
destil.	*destilla* (distill); *destillatus* (distilled)
det.	detect; detection; detergent; determine; detour; detritus; *detur* (let it be given)
detox.	detoxicate; detoxication; detoxify
Dex.	Dexamethasone
DEXA	Dexamethasone
DF	damage free; dead fetus; deficiency factor; dorsi-flexion
DFA	direct fluorescent antibody
DFDT	di-fluoro-diphenyl-trichloroethane
DFE	distal femoral epiphysis
DFMO	di-fluoro-methyl-ornithine
DFMR	daily fetal movement recording
DFO	Deferoxamine

DFP	diastolic filling pressure; diisopropyl-fluoro-phosphate
DFS	disease-free survival
DFU	dead fetus in utero; dideoxy-fluoro-uridine
dg	deci-gram
DG	deoxy-glucose; deoxy-guanosine; diagnosis; diastolic gallop di-glyceride; disto-gingival
DGDP	deoxy-guanosine di-phosphate
DGI	disseminated gonococcal infection
DGMP	deoxy-guanosine mono-phosphate
DGTP	deoxy-guanosine tri-phosphate
DH	delayed hypersensitivity; diaphragmatic hernia
DHA	di-hydro-alanine; di-hydroxy-acetone
DHAD	di-hydroxy-anthracene-dione
DHAP	di-hydroxy-acetone phosphate
DHAS	de-hydroepi-androsterone sulfate
DHBV	duck hepatitis B virus
DHEA	de-hydro-epi-androsterone
DHEAS	de-hydro-epi-androsterone sulfate
DHF	dengue hemorrhagic fever
DHFR	di-hydro-folate reductase
D.Hg.	Doctor of Hygiene
DHL	diffuse histiocytic lymphoma
DHMA	di-hydroxy-mandelic acid
DHPMG	di-hydroxy-propoxy-methyl guanine
DHR	delayed hypersensitivity reaction
DHS	delayed hyper-sensitivity
DHSR	delayed hyper-sensitivity reaction
DHST	delayed hypersensitivity to skin testing
DHT	di-hydro-tachysterol; di-hydro-testosterone
D.Hy.	Doctor of Hygiene
DI	diabetes insipidus; diagnostic imaging
dia.	diameter
diag.	diagnose; diagnosis; diagnostic; diagonal; diagram
diam.	diameter
DIAR	Dextran-induced anaphylactoid reaction
DIC	diffuse intravascular coagulation; Dimethyl-Imidazole-Carboxyamide (Dacarbazine); disseminated intravascular clotting; disseminated intravascular coagulation
d.i.d.	*detur in duplo* (let it be given twice)
DID	drug-induced diarrhea
DIDMOAD	Diabetes Insipidus, Diabetes Mellitus, Optic Atrophy, Deafness

dieb. alt.	*diebus alternis* (on alternate days)
dieb. tert.	*diebus tertiis* (every third day)
DIEM	died in emergency room
DIFF	difference; different; differential
dig.	*digeratur* (let it be digested); digitalis; digitoxin; digoxin
digit.	*digitus* (digit; finger)
dil.	dilate (expand; stretch); *dilue* (dilute)
DILD	diffuse infiltrative lung disease
DILE	drug-induced lupus erythematosus
diluc.	*diluculo* (at daybreak)
dilut.	*dilutus* (diluted)
dim.	*dimidius* (one-half)
DIM	divalent ion metabolism
DIP	desquamative interstitial pneumonitis; Dual In-line Package; distal inter-phalangeal
d.i.p.a.	*divide in partes aequales* (divide into equal parts)
DIPJ	distal inter-phalangeal joint
dir.	*directione* (directions)
dir. prop.	*directione propria* (with proper direction)
disc.	discontinue; discontinued
disch.	discharge; discharged
DISH	diffuse idiopathic skeletal hyperostosis
DISI	dorsiflexed intercalated segment instability
disl.	dislocation
disp.	dispense; disperse; dispireme
dist.	*distilla* (distill); distilled; district
DIT	diet-induced thermogenesis; di-iodo-tyrosine
div.	*divide* (divide); division
DJD	degenerative joint disease
DK	dark; diseased kidney
DKA	diabetic keto-acidosis
DKB	deep knee bends
dl	deci-liter (deci-litre)
dL	deci-liter (deci-litre)
DL	day-light; difference lumen; diffusing capacity of lung; direct line; direct link; disto-lingual; disto-labial; Donath-Landsteiner (test); Doxorubicin, Lomustine
DLE	discoid lupus erythematosus; disseminated lupus erythematosus
DLI	disto-labio-incisal; disto-linguo-incisal
DLO	disto-linguo-occlusal

DLP	disto-linguo-pulpal
DLR	Detection Limit for Reporting Purposes
dm	deci-meter (deci-metre)
dM	deci-morgan
DM	diabetes mellitus; diastolic murmur; digital machine; direct memory; distant metastasis; Dopamine; double minute
DMA	di-methoxy-amphetamine; Direct Memory Access
DMAC	disseminated mycobacterium avium complex
DMARD	disease modifying anti-rheumatic drug
DMCT	de-methyl-chlor-tetracycline
D.M.D.	Doctor of Dental Medicine
DMD	Duchenne's Muscular Dystrophy
DME	durable medical equipment
DMERC	durable medical equipment regional carrier
DMF	decayed, missing, filled; di-methyl-formamide
DMFS	decayed, missing, filled surfaces
DMHLL	diffuse mixed histiocytic-lymphocytic lymphoma
DMI	diaphragmatic myocardial infarction
DML	diffuse mixed lymphoma
DMM	des-methyl-misonidazole; di-methyl-myleran
DMN	di-methyl-nitrosamine
DMO	Di-methadi-one
DMPA	depo-medroxy-progesterone acetate
DMPP	di-methyl-phenyl-piperazinium
D.M.R.D.	Diploma in Medical Radio-Diagnosis (British)
D.M.R.T.	Diploma in Medical Radio-Therapy (British)
DMSA-RS	di-mercapto-succinic acid renal scan
DMSO	di-methyl sulf-oxide
DMT	di-methyl-tryptamine
DMTT	di-methyl-thionotetrahydro-thiadiazine (Dazomet)
DN	Deci-nem; dextrose to nitrogen ratio; dibucaine number
DNA	deoxyribo-nucleic acid; did not answer; did not apply; do not apply
DNAP	Dinosam
DNase	deoxyribo-nucle-ase
DNB	di-nitro-benzene
DNBP	Dinoseb
DNC	di-nitro-carbanilide; di-nitro-cresol
DNCB	di-nitro-chloro-benzene
DND	died — natural death
DNFB	di-nitro-fluoro-benzene

DNJ	deoxy-no-jirimycin
DNOC	di-nitro-o-cresol (Antinonin; Dinitrol; Ditrosol; Sinox)
DNOCHP	Dinex
DNOSAP	Dinosam
DNOSBP	Dinoseb
DNP	deoxyribo-nucleo-protein
DNPH	di-nitro-phenyl-hydrazine
DNPM	di-nitro-phenyl-morphine
DNR	Dau-no-rubicin; did not receive; do not resuscitate
D/NS	dextrose in normal saline
DNS	Dansyl; did not show; dysplastic nervus syndrome
DNSAP	Dinosam
DNSBP	Dinoseb
D.N.Sc.	Doctor of Nursing Science
DNT	did not test; do not test; do not touch; do not turn
DO	oxygen delivery
D.O.	Doctor of Osteopathy; doctor's orders
DO	diamine oxidase; disto-occlusal; delivery of oxygen
DOA	date of adjustment; date of admission; date of arrival; dead on arrival
DOAP	Daunorubicin, Oncovin, Ara-C, Prednisone
DOB	date of birth
DOC	date of conception; died of other causes; de-oxy-cholate; doctor
DOCA	de-oxy-corticosterone acetate
DOCs	de-oxy-corticoids
DOD	date of death; died of disease; drug over-dose; dodecylguanidine (Dodine)
DOE	date of examination; dyspnea on exercise; dyspnea on exertion
DOMA	dihydr-oxy-mandelic acid; dimeth-oxy-methyl-amphetamine
DON	determination of need; diazo-oxo-norleucine
DOOR	deafness, oncyhodystrophy, osteodystrophy, retardation
DOPA	dihydr-oxy-phenyl-alanine
DOPAC	dihydr-oxy-phenyl-acetic acid
DOS	disk operating system
DOT	daily observed therapy
Dox.	Doxorubicin
DOXO	Doxorubicin
DOX-PT	Doxorubicin, Platinol
D.P.	Doctor of Pharmacy; Doctor of Podiatry

DP	data processing; data processor; diastolic pressure; direct pressure; direct puncture; distal phalanx; disto-pulpal; dorsalis pedis; dorsi-palmar
DPA	di-propyl-acetate
DPC	delayed primary closure; distal palmar crease
DPD	diffuse pulmonary disease
DPDLL	diffuse poorly differentiated lymphocytic lymphoma
DPG	di-phospho-glycerate; displacement placento-gram
D.P.H.	Department of Public Health; Doctor of Public Health
DPL	disto-pulpo-lingual; disto-pulpo-labial
DPL$_{ab}$	disto-pulpo-labial
DPL$_{in}$	disto-pulpo-lingual
D.P.M.	Doctor of Podiatric Medicine
DPN	diphospho-pyridine nucleotide
DPP	dimethoxy-phenyl penicillin
DPS	dimethyl-poly-siloxane; Diversified Pharmaceutical Services
DPT	Demerol, Phenergan, Thorazine; Diphtheria, Pertussis, and Tetanus; di-propyl-tryptamine
DPTI	diastolic pressure-time index
DPTV	Diphtheria, Pertussis, and Tetanus Vaccine
DPVNS	diffuse pigmented villo-nodular synovitis
Dr	debit (bookkeeping abbreviation); doctor; door; drive; driver
DR	deep reflex; deep reflexes; degeneration reaction; delivery room; diabetic retinopathy; diagnostic radiology; doctor; door; drive; driver
DRAs	Dextran-reactive antibodies
DRE	digital rectal examination
DREZ	dorsal root entry zone
DRF	dose-reduction factor
DRG	diagnosis-related group
Dr.P.H.	Doctor of Public Health
drs.	dressing
DRS	disease-free survival
drsg.	dressing
DRTA	distal renal tubular acidosis
d.s.	*debita spissitudine* (of the proper consistency)
D/S	dextrose in saline
DS	dehydro-epiandrosterone sulfate; dextrose-saline; double strength; double-stranded; Down's syndrome
DSA	digital subtraction angiography

DSAG	digital subtraction angio-graphy
DSAP	disseminated superficial actinic porokeratosis
DSAS	discrete sub-aortic stenosis
D.Sc.	Doctor of Science
D.S.C.	Doctor or Surgical Chiropody
DSD	dry sterile dressing
DSEC	digital subtraction echo-cardiogram
DSECG	digital subtraction echo-cardio-gram
DSI	digital subtraction imaging
DSM	dextrose solution mixture; Diagnostic and Statistical Manual of Mental Disorders
DSP	Digital Signal Processing
DSPN	digital symmetric peripheral neuropathy
DSR	dynamic (three-dimensional) spatial reconstructor
DST	Dexamethasone suppression test; donor specific transfusion
D-stix	Dextro-stix
DSVP	down-stream venous pressure
DT	day-time; delay time; delirium tremens; deoxy-thymidine; digital time; diphtheria toxoid; diphtheria, tetanus; double time; duration tetany; dye test
DTAFFB	descending thoracic aorto-femoral femoral-bypass
DTBC	d-tubo-curarine (Curare; tubo-curarine chloride)
DTC	d-tubo-curarine (Curare; tubo-curarine chloride)
d. t. d.	*datur talis dosis* (give a such a dose); *dentur tales doses* (give a such a dose)
DTDP	deoxy-thymidine di-phosphate
2D-TEEC	2-dimensional trans-esophageal echo-cardiography
DTF	detector transfer function
DTH	delayed-type hypersensitivity
DTHS	delayed-type hyper-sensitivity
DTI	dipryridamole-thallium imaging
DTIC	Dimethyl-Triazeno-Imidazole-Carboxyamide (Dacarbazine)
DTM	deoxy-thymidine monophosphate; dermatophyte test medium
DTN	diphtheria toxin normal
DTNBA	di-thiobis-nitro-benzoic acid
DTP	Diphtheria, Tetanus, and Pertussis; distal tingling on percussion
DTPA	diethylene-triamine penta-acetic acid (pentetic acid)
DTPV	Diphtheria, Tetanus, and Pertussis Vaccine

DTR	deep tendon reflex; dietetic technician registered
DTRs	deep tendon reflexes
DTs	delirium tremens
DTS	donor-specific transfusion
DTT	diphtheria-tetanus-toxoid; di-thio-threitol
DTZ	Dia-tri-zoate
DU	deoxy-uridine; duodenal ulcer
DUB	dysfunctional uterine bleeding
DUF	Doppler Ultrasonic Flowmeter
DUI	driving under influence
DUII	driving under influence of intoxicants
DUIL	driving under influence of liquor
DUL	diffuse undifferentiated lymphoma
DUMP	deoxy-uridine mono-phosphate
DUNHL	diffuse undifferentiated non-Hodgkin's lymphoma
duod.	duodenum
DUP	decubitus ulcer potential; duplicate; duplication
DUR-1	distal ureter resection — unilateral
DUR-2	distal ureter resection — bilateral
dur. dol.	*durante dolore* (while pain lasts)
DUSN	diffuse unilateral subacute neuroretinitis
DUTP	deoxy-uridine tri-phosphate
D&V	diarrhea and vomiting
DV	double variations; double vision; dual valve
DVA	distance visual acuity
DVD	dissociated vertical deviation; dissociated vertical divergence
DVI	digital vascular imaging
DVIU	direct vision internal urethrotomy
D.V.M.	Doctor of Veterinary Medicine
DVM	digital volt-meter
D.V.M.S.	Doctor of Veterinary Medicine and Surgery
DVP-Asp	Daunorubicin, Vincristine, Prednisone, Asparaginase
D.V.S.	Doctor of Veterinary Science; Doctor of Veterinary Surgery
DVSA	digital venous subtraction angiography
DVSAG	digital venous subtraction angio-graphy
DVT	deep vein thrombosis; deep venous thrombosis
DVTSP	deep venous thrombus scinti-photography
D/W	dextrose in water; distilled water
DW	dead-weight; dextrose in water; distilled water
5DW	5% dextrose in water

D5W	5% dextrose in water
DWD	died without disease; diffuse well-differentiated
DWDLL	diffuse well-differentiated lymphocytic leukemia
DWI	driving while intoxicated
DX	Dextran; diagnosis; distance
DXM	Dexamethasone
DXRT	deep X-Ray therapy
dy.	delivery
Dy	Dysprosium
DYSZ	dyszooamylia; dyszoospermia
DZ	dizygotic; dizzy; dizziness; dozen

～ E ～

εACA	epsilon-amino-caproic acid
e	electron; natural logarithm base (e = 2.718281828459...)
e⁺	positron (positive charge)
e⁻	electron (negative charge); the heavy chain of IgE
E	ear; east; edema; Einstein; Einsteinium; electric charge; electric; electron; emergency; emmetropia; empty; end; energy; *Entamoeba*; enzyme; epinephrine; error; *Escherichia*; esophoria; Etoposide; Europe; European; excellent; eye
E_1	estrone
E_2	estradiol
E_3	estriol
E_4	estetrol
ea.	each
EA	early antigen; erythrocyte antibody; ethacrynic acid
EAA	excitatory amino acid
EAb	elective abortion
EAB	elective abortion
EAC	Ehrlich ascites carcinoma; erythrocyte-antibody complement; external auditory canal
E-ACA	epsilon-amino-caproic acid
ead.	*eadem* (same)
EAEM	experimental allergic encephalo-myelitis
EAHF	eczema, asthma, hay fever
EAHLG	equine anti-human lymphoblast globulin
EAHLS	equine anti-human lymphoblast serum
EAM	external auditory meatus
EAN	experimental allergic neuritis
EAP	Etoposide, Adriamycin, Platinol; epi-allo-pregnenolone
EA-ST	Emory Angioplasty versus Surgery Trial
EB	elementary body; epidermolysis-bullosa; Epstein-Barr
EBDA	effective balloon-dilated area
EBF	erythro-blastosis fetalis

EBI	emetine-bismuth-iodide
EBL	erythro-blastic leukemia; estimated blood loss
EBNA	Epstein-Barr nuclear antigen
EBT	external beam therapy
EBV	Epstein-Barr virus
EBV-B	Epstein-Barr virus-transformed B-cells
EC	effective circulation; ejection click; enteric coated; error corrected (bookkeeping abbreviation); *Escherichia coli*; extra-cellular
ECA	etha-crynic acid; external carotid artery
E-CABG	endarterectomy and coronary artery bypass graft
E-CAT	emission computer-assisted tomography
ECBO	enteric cytopathogenic bovine orphan (virus)
ECBV	effective circulating blood volume
ECC	edema, clubbing, cyanosis; emergency cardiac care; emergency cardiac compression; endo-cervical curettage; external cardiac compression; extra-cellular compartment; extra-corporeal circulation
ECCD	endo-cardial cushion defect
ECCE	extra-capsular cataract extract
ECD	endocardial cushion defect
ECDO virus	enteric cytopathogenic dog orphan virus
ECF	effective capillary flow; eosinophil chemotactic factor; extended care facility; extra-cellular fluid
ECF-A	eosinophil chemotactic factor of anaphylaxis
ECFV	extra-cellular fluid volume
ECG	electro-cardio-gram; electro-cardio-graphy; electro-cortico-gram
ECHO	Enteric Cytopathogenic Human Orphan (virus)
ECHO-C	echo-cardiogram; echo-cardiography
ECI	electro-cerebral inactivity
ECIB	extra-corporeal irradiation of blood
EC-IC	extra-cranial — intra-cranial
ECIL	extra-corporeal irradiation of lymph
ECLAM	endothelial cell leukocyte adhesion molecule
ECLT	euglobulin clot lysis time
ECM	erythema chronicum migrans; extra-cellular material
ECMO	extra-corporeal membrane oxygenation
ECMO virus	enteric cytopathogenic monkey orphan virus
ECoG	electro-cortico-gram; electro-cortico-graphy
ECOG	Eastern Cooperative Oncology Group
E. coli	*Escherichia coli*

ECRB	extensor carpi radialis brevis
ECRL	extensor carpi radialis longus
ECS	electro-cerebral silence; electro-convulsive shock; electronic claim submission; extra-cellular space
ECSO virus	enteric cytopathogenic swine orphan virus
ECSWL	extra-corporeal shock-wave lithotripsy
ECT	electro-convulsive therapy; emission computed tomography; emission computerized tomography; euglobulin clot test
ECU	extensor carpi ulnaris
ECV	extra-cellular volume
ECW	extra-cellular water
ED	ear disease; effective dose; Ehlers-Danlos (syndrome); Emergency Department; end-diastolic; epileptiform discharge; erythema dose; extensive disease; eye desease
ED_{50}	effective dose — 50%
EDA	elbow dis-articulation; ethylene-di-amine
EDB	ethylene di-bromide; extensor digitorum brevis
EDC	estimated date of conception; estimated date of confinement; expected date of conception; expected date of confinement; extensor digitorum communis
EDD	estimated date of delivery; expected date of delivery
EDF	eosinophil differentiation factor
EDL	end-diastolic length; extensor digitorum longus
EDP	end-diastolic pressure
EDQ	extensor digiti quinti
EDR	effective direct radiation; electro-dermal response
EDRF	endothelium-derived relaxing factor
EDS	Ehlers-Danlos syndrome; excessive daytime sleepiness
EDTA	ethylene-diamine-tetraacetic acid
EDV	end-diastolic volume
EDVI	end-diastolic volume index
EDX	electro-diagnosis
EE	equine encephalitis; eye and ear
EEA	electro-encephalic audiometry; energy experience of activity
EEDC synd.	ectrodactyl-ectodermal dysplasia-clefting syndrome
EEE	Eastern equine encephalomyelitis (virus)
EEEP	end-expiratory esophageal pressure
EEG	electro-encephalo-gram; electro-encephalo-graphy
EENT	eye, ear, nose, throat

EER	electro-encephalic response
EERP	extended endocardial resection procedure
EES	erythromycin ethyl-succinate
EF	ectopic focus; ejection fraction; extended field
EFAs	essential fatty acids
EFC	endogenous fecal calcium
EFE	endocardial fibro-elastosis
Eff.	effective; effervescent (tablet)
EFM	electronic fetal monitoring
EFV	extracellular fluid volume
EFVC	expiratory flow-volume curve
EFW	estimated fetal weight
e.g.	*exempli gratia* (for example)
EG	esophago-gastrectomy; esophago-gastric
EGA	estimated gestational age
EGB	eosinophilic granuloma of bone
EGC	early gastric cancer
EGD	esophago-gastro-duodenoscopy
EGF	epidermal growth factor
EGFR	epidermal growth factor receptor
EGG	electro-gastro-gram
EGJ	esophago-gastric junction
EGL	eosinophilic granuloma of lung
EGOT	erythrocyte glutamatic oxaloacetic transaminase
EGS	electro-galvanic stimulation
EGTA	esophageal gastric tube airway
EH	enlarged heart; essential hypertension
EHB	elevated head of bed
EHBD	extra-hepatic biliary duct
EHBF	estimated hepatic blood flow; exercise hyperemia blood flow
EHC	entero-hepatic circulation; essential hyper-cholesterolemia
EHD	epizootic hemorrhagic disease
EHEC	entero-hemorrhagic *Escherichia coli*
EHF	epidemic hemorrhagic fever; exophthalamus hyperthyroid factor
EHL	effective half-life; endogenous hyper-lipidemia; extensor hallucis longus
EHO	extra-hepatic obstruction
EHT	essential hyper-tension
E/I	expiration / inspiration (ratio)

EI	enzyme inhibitor; eosinophilic index
EIA	electro-immuno-assay; enzyme immuno-assay
EIAL	exercise-induced airflow limitation
EIAV	equine infectious anemia virus
EID	electro-immuno-diffusion; Emergency Infusion Device
EIEC	entero-invasive *Escherichia coli*
EIN	endometrial intraepithelial neoplasia
EINI	elective inguinal node irradiation
EIP	extensor indicis proprius
EIPV	Enhanced-potency Inactivated Poliovirus Vaccine
EIS	Epidemic Intelligence Service
EIT	erythrocyte iron turnover
EJ	elbow jerk
EJN	external jugular vein
ejus.	*ejusdem* (of the same)
EKC	epidemic kerato-conjunctivitis
EKG	electro-cardio-gram; electro-kardio-gram (German: kardio = heart; gramma = mark); electro-cardio-graph; electro-kardio-graph (German: kardio = heart; grapein = to write)
EKyG	electro-kymo-gram
EL	electro-leukemia
ELAM	endothelial (cell) leukocyte adhesion molecule
ELAS	extended lymph-adenopathy syndrome
elec.	election; elective; electric; electrical; electricity; electron
elem.	element; elementary
elev.	elevate; elevated; elevation
ELIEDA	enzyme-linked immuno-electro-diffusion assay
ELISA	enzyme-linked immuno-sorbent assay
ELIX	elixir (from Arabic: al-iksir)
ELSS	extravehicular life support system
ELT	euglobulin lysis time
EM	ejection murmur; electro-magnetic; electron microscope; emergency medicine; emmetropia; erythema migrans
EMA	epithelial membrane antigen
EMA-CF	Etoposide, Methotrexate, Adriamycin, Citrovorum Factor
E-mail	electronic mail
EMB	endo-myocardial biopsy; eosin methylene blue
EMC	encephalo-myo-carditis
EMD	electro-mechanical dissociation; electro-myocardial dissociation

EMF	electro-magnetic flowmeter; electro-magnetic force; electro-motive force; endo-myocardial fibrosis; eosinophil maturation factor; erythrocyte maturation factor
EMG	electro-myelo-gram; electro-myo-gram; electro-myo-graphy; exophthalamus macroglossia gigantism
EMI	electro-magnetic interference
EMIT	enzyme-multiplied immunoassay technique
EMLA	eutectic mixture of local anesthetics
e.m.p.	*ex modo praescripto* (as prescribed)
emp.	*emplastrum* (a plaster)
EMR	electro-magnetic radiation
E.M.S.	Emergency Medical Service (British)
EMS	eosinophilia myalgia syndrome
EMSU	early morning specimen of urine
EMT	Emergency Medical Technician
e.m.u.	electro-magnetic units
emul.	emulate; emulation; emulsify; *emulsio* (emulsion)
EMW	electro-magnetic wave; electro-magnetic waves
EN	erythema nodosum; eye nerve
ENA	Emergency Nurses Association; extractable nuclear antigen
ENE	ethyl-nor-epinephrine
ENG	electro-neurography; electro-nystagmo-gram electro-nystagmo-graphy; English; engineer; engineering
ENGR	engineer; engineering
ENL	erythema nodosum leprosum
ENT	ear, nose, throat
EO	ear operation; ethylene oxide; even and odd; extra oil; eye operation; eyes opened
EOA	esophageal obturator airway
E&OE	errors and omissions expected
EOE	ethiodized oil emulsion
EOG	electro-oculo-gram; electro-olfacto-gram
EOM	end of message; end of month; extra-ocular movement; extra-ocular muscles
EOMB	explanation of Medicare benefits
EOMI	extra-ocular movement intact; extra-ocular muscles intact
EOP	external occipital protuberance
E.O.R.T.C.	European Organization for Radiation Therapy in Cancer

eos.	eosinophil; eosinophils
eosin.	eosinophil; eosinophils
EOT	effective oxygen transport; end of text; end of transmission
EP	ectopic pregnancy; electro-phoresis; endogenous pyrogen; erythrocyte protoporphyrin; erythro-poietin; evoked potential
EPA	eicosa-pentaenoic acid; Environmental Protection Agency
EPAP	expiratory positive airway pressure
EPB	extensor pollicis brevis
EPBF	effective pulmonary blood flow
EPC	epilepsia partialis continua
EPDT	early pregnancy detection test
EPEC	entero-pathogenic *Escherichia coli*
EPF	early pregnancy factor; eosinophilic pustular folliculitis; exophthalmus producing factor
epi.	epinephrine; episiotomy; epithelial
EPIN	epinephrine
epis.	*epistomium* (a stopper)
EPIS	episiotomy
epith.	ephithalaxia; epithalamus; epithelial; epithelium
EPL	extensor pollicis longus
EPM	electronic pace-maker
EPMR	electron para-magnetic resonance
EPP	end-plate potential; erythropoietic proto-porphyria
EPPL	epithelial, possibly precancerous lesion
EPPP	erythro-poietic proto-porphyria
EPR	electro-phrenic respiration; electron paramagnetic resonance; epitym-panic recess; estradiol production rate
EPS	electro-pyhsiologic study; exophthalamus producing substance; express prostatic secretion; extra-pyramidal signs; extra-pyramidal symptoms
EPSDT	early periodic screening diagnosis and treatment
EPSP	excitatory post-synaptic potential
EPTD	extra-polated total dose
EPTFE	expanded poly-tetra-fluoro-ethylene
eq.	equal; equation; equivalent
equiv.	equivalent
Er	Erbium; error corrected (bookkeeping abbreviation)
E/R	external rotation

ER	early response; ejection rate; electric response; Emergency Room; endoplasmic reticulum; error corrected (bookkeeping abbreviation); estrogen receptor; evoked response; expiratory reserve; external resistance; external rotation
ERA	electric response audiometry; estroadiol receptor assay; estrogen receptor assay; evoked response audiometry
ERBD	endoscopic retrograde biliary drainage
ERBF	effective renal blood flow
ERC	erythropoietic responsive cell
ERCP	endoscopic retrograde cholangio-pancreatography
ERCPG	endoscopic retrograde cholangio-pancreato-graphy
ER&F	external reduction and fixation
ERF	Education and Research Foundation; external reduction and fixation
ERG	electro-retino-gram
ERIA	electro-radio-immuno-assay
ERICA	enzyme-linked immuno-chemical assay; estrogen receptor immuno-cytochemical assay
ERISA	Employee Retirement Income Security Act
ERP	effective refractory period; equine rhino-pneumonitis; estrogen receptor protein
ERPF	effective renal plasma flow
ERS	endoscopic retrograde sphincterotomy
ERT	estrogen replacement therapy
ERUS	endo-rectal ultra-sound
ERV	expiratory reserve volume
Es	Einsteinium
ES	ear surgery; early sign; early signal; early sound; early stage; ejection signal; ejection stage; emergency surgery; eye surgery
ESB	electrical stimulation to brain
Esc.	escape; *Escherichia*
E.S.C.	European Society of Cardiology
ESD	early-stage diagnosis
ESEP	extreme somatosensory evoked potential
ESF	erythropoietic-stimulating factor
ESL	end-systolic length
ESM	ejection-systolic murmur
eso.	esophagoscopy; esophagus
esp.	especially; espundia
ESP	end-systolic pressure; eosinophil stimulation promoter; extra-sensory perception

ESR	electron spin resonance; erythrocyte sedimentation rate
ESRD	end-stage renal disease
ess.	essential
ESS	erythrocyte sensitizing substance
ESSEP	extreme somato-sensory evoked potential
est.	established (patient)
EST	Eastern Standard Time; electro-shock therapy; electro-shock treatment
e.s.u.	electro-static unit
ESV	end-systolic volume
ESVI	end-systolic volume index
ESWL	extracorporeal shock-wave lithotripsy
et	*et* (and)
Et.	ethyl; etiology
ET	effective temperature; effective time; ejection time; endotracheal tube; enterically transmitted; eustachian tube
ETA	estimated time of activity; estimated time of arrival; 2-ethyliso-thionicotin-amide (Amidazine; Ethionamide)
ETAF	epithelial thymic activating factor
et al.	*et alii* (and others)
etc.	*et cetera* (and so on)
ETD	extrapolated total dose
ETEC	entero-toxic *Escherichia coli*
ETF	eustachian tube function
ETH	elixir terpin hydrate
ETH/C	elixir terpin hydrate with Codeine
ETKM	Every Test Known to Man
ETM	Erythromycin (Erycin; Erythrocin; Ilotycin; Retcin)
Et$_2$O	ether
ETOE	efficiency of tissue oxygen extraction
EtOH	ethanol; ethyl alcohol
ETP	eustachian tube pressure
ETS	environmental tobacco smoke
ETT	esophageal transit time; exercise tolerance test; extra-thyroidal thyroxine
ETU	Emergency and Trauma Unit
Eu	Europe; Europium
EU	Ehrlich unit; endotoxin unit; enzyme unit; Europe
EUA	examination under anesthesia
eV	electron volt
EV	epidermodysplasia verruciformis; extra-vascular

EVA	Etoposide, Vincristine, Adriamycin
evac.	evacuate; evacuated; evacuation
eval.	evaluate; evaluated; evaluation
evap.	evaporation
EVAP	Etoposide, Vinblastine, Ara-C, Platinol
EVLW	extra-vascular lung water
EVR	endocardial viability ratio
EVS	elective variceal sclerosis; endoscopic variceal sclerotherapy
EVST	endoscopic variceal sclero-therapy
EW	elsewhere; emergency ward; eye-wash
EWB	estrogen withdrawal bleeding
EWL	egg-white lysozyme
EX	examination; exception; exercise
exam	examination
exc.	excision; exception; exclude; exclusion
EXEC	executive
ExHBF	exercise hyperemia blood flow
exhib.	*exhibeatur* (let it be given); exhibit; exhibition
Ex MO	express money order (bookkeeping abbreviation)
EXP	expand; expect; expectorate; expel; experiment; expiration; expired; exploration; explore; expose; exposition; exposure
expec.	expectancy; expectant; expectation; expectorant; expectorate; expectoration
exper.	experiment
exp. lap.	exploratory laparotomy
expt.	experiment
exptl.	experimental
ext.	extend; *extende* (extend; spread); extension; exterior; external; extract; extraction; *extractum* (extract)
extn.	extension
ext. rot.	external rotation
ExUG	excretory uro-gram

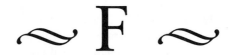

f.	*fiat* (let it be done); focal length; frequency
F	face; factor; Fahrenheit; fair; false; fan; fangus; farad; faraday; fast; fat; fatal; father; February; feces; feet; female; fertility; fetus; fever; field; Filaria; film; finger; fish; flat; flatus; flea; fluorine; fly; foot; force; formula; French; frequency; Friday; frog; full; fusiformis
F$_1$	filial — first generation
F$_2$	filial — second generation
F-12	Freon 12
FA	false aneurysm; father; fatty acid; femoral artery; first aid; fluorescent antibody; folic acid; fore-arm; free acid
FAB	formalin ammonium bromide; fragment antigen binding
FABF	fore-arm blood flow
FAC	Federal Allowable Cost; Fluorouracil, Adriamycin, Cyclophosphamide
FACA	Fellow of the American College of Anesthesiologists
FACD	Fellow of the American College of Dentists
FACOG	Fellow of the American College of Obstetricians and Gynecologists
FACP	Fellow of the American College of Physicians
FACR	Fellow of the American College of Radiologists
FACS	Fellow of the American College of Surgeons; fluorescence activated cell sorter
FACSM	Fellow of the American College of Sports Medicine
FAC-XRT	Fluorouracil, Adriamycin, Cytoxan — Radiation Therapy
FAD	flavin adenine dinucleotide
FADF	flourescent antibody dark field
Fahr.	Fahrenheit
FAI	functional aerobic impairment
F-AIDS	Feline — Auto Immune Deficiency Syndrome
Fam.	family
FAM	Fluorouracil, Adriamycin, Mitomycin C
FAMA	fluorescent antibody to membrane antigen

FAMe	Fluorouracil, Adriamycin, MeCCNU
FAMS	Fluorouracil, Adriamycin, Mitomycin, Streptozotocin
FANA	fluorescent anti-nuclear antibody
FAO	Food and Agriculture Organization (of the United Nations)
FAP	familial adenomatous polyposis; fibrillating action potential; Fluorouracil, Adriamycin, Platinol
fasc.	*fasciculus* (bundle)
FAST	fluoro-allergo-sorbent test
FAT	Fetal Activity Test; first-aid kit; fluorescent antibody test; 5-Flourouracil, Adriamycin, Trazinate
FATS	familial atherosclerosis treatment study
FAV	feline ataxia virus
FAX	facsimile (transmission or reproduction via telephone line)
FB	finger breadth; fluid balance; food bank; foreign body; frog belly; frontal bone
FBD	functional bowel disorder
FBE	full blood examination
FBF	forearm blood flow
FBI	Federal Bureau of Investigation
FBOA	Fellow of the British Optical Association
FBP	femoral blood pressure; fibrinogen breakdown products
FBS	fasting blood sugar; fetal bovine serum
FC	finger clubbing; Foley catheter; food chain
FCA	ferritin conjugated antibody; Freund's complete adjuvant
FCAP	Fellow of the College of American Pathologists
FCB	folli-cultis barbae (tinea barbae)
FCC	Federal Communications Commission
FCCP	Fellow of the American College of Chest Physicians
FCIF	fixed cell immune fluorescence
FCP	Fellow of the College of Physicians; Fluorouracil, Cytoxan, Prednisone
FCR	flexor carpi radialis
FCS	Fellow of the Chemical Society
FCU	flexor carpi ulnaris
f.d.	*febre durante* (while the fever lasts); *fracta dosi* (in divided doses)
FD	Fabry's disease; fatal dose; feline distemper; filing date; Fire Department; focal distance; forceps delivery
FD_{50}	fatal dose — 50%
FDA	fronto-dextra anterior (position of fetus); Food and Drug Administration

FDB	first-degree burn; flexor digitorum brevis
FDC	follicular dendritic cell
FDG	flouro-deoxy-glucose
FDHS	first-degree heart sound
FDL	flexor digitorum longus
FDNS	familial dysplastic nevus syndrome
FDP	fibrin degradation products; flexor digitorum profundus; fronto-dextra posterior (position of fetus)
FDQ	flexor digiti quinti
FDS	flexor digitorum sublimis; flexor digitorum superficialis
FDT	fronto-dextra transversa (position of fetus)
FDUMP	fluoro-deoxy-uridine mono-phosphate
Fe	February; female; *ferrum* (iron)
FE	feline enteritis
Fe^{2+}	ferrous
Fe^{3+}	ferric
Feb.	February
FEC	forced expiratory capacity
FECFV	functional extra-cellular fluid volume
FECG	fetal electro-cardio-gram; fetal electro-cardio-graphy
$FeCO_3$	ferrous-carbonate
FECP	free erythrocyte copro-porphyria
fe. cult.	fecal culture
FECV	functional extra-cellular (fluid) volume
FEF	forced expiratory flow
FEF_{max}	forced expiratory flow — maximum
FEKG	fetal electro-kardio-gram (fetal electro-cardio-gram)
FELH	familial erythrophagocytic lympho-histiocytosis
FeLV	feline leukemia virus
FEM	female; femoral; femur
fem. int.	*femoribus internus* (at the inner side of the thighs)
F.E.M.S.	Federation of European Microbiologists' Societies
FENa	fractional excretion of natrium (*natrium* = sodium)
Fe_2O_3	ferric-oxide
$Fe(OH)_3$	ferric-hydroxide
FEP	fluorinated ethylene propylene; free erythrocyte porphyrin
FEPP	free erythrocyte proto-porphyrin
ferv.	*fervens* (boiling)
FESg	forced expiratory spiro-gram
$FeSO_4$	ferrous-sulfate
FESS	functional endoscopic sinus surgery
FET	field-effective transistor; forced expiratory technique; forced expiratory time

FEV	forced expiratory volume
FEV$_1$	forced expiratory volume in one second
ff.	following
FF	fat free; fecal frequency; fertility factor; filtration fraction; frog face
FFA	fluorescein fundoscopy and angiography; free fatty acid
FFC	fixed flexion contracture; free from chlorine
FFD	fat-free diagnosis; final filing date; focal film distance
FFDCA	Federal Food, Drug and Cosmetic Act
FFM	fat-free mass
FFP	fresh frozen plasma
FFPS	Fellow of the Faculty of Physicians and Surgeons
FFR	freedom from relapse
FF-RF	full-fledged risk factor
FFS	failure-free survival
FFT	finger-finger test; flicker fusion test; flicker fusion threshold
FFW	fat-free weight
FGD	fatal granulomatous disease
FGF	fibroblast growth factor
f.h.	*fiat hasutus* (let a draught be made)
FH	facies hepatica; family history; fetal hand; fetal head; fetal heart
FHC	facies hippo-cratica
FHF	fulminant hepatic failure
FHH	familial hypocalciuric hypercalcemia
FHL	flexor hallucis longus
FHR	fetal heart rate
FHS	fetal heart sound
FHT	fetal heart tone
f.i.	*femoribus internus* (at the inner side of the thighs)
FI	feline influenza; finger infection; forced inspiration
FIA	fluoro-immuno-assay; Freund's incomplete adjuvant
Fial.	fialuridine
FICD	Fellow of the International College of Dentists
FICO$_2$	fraction of inspired carbon dioxide
FICS	Fellow of the International College of Surgeons
FID	flame ionization detector
FIF	fetus in fetu; forced inspiratory flow
FIFO	First In, First Out
FIGA	form-imino-glutamic acid

FIGEP	field inversion gel electro-phoresis
FIH	first intention healing
filt.	*filtra* (filter)
FIO	free in and out
FIO$_2$	forced inspiratory oxygen; fractional inspired oxygen
FIPV	feline infectious peritonitis virus
FIVC	forced inspiratory vital capacity
FJN	familial juvenile nephrophthisis
FJP	familial juvenile polyposis
fl.	*fluidus* (fluid)
FL	facies leontina; filtration leukapheresis; focal lesion
f.l.a.	*fiat lege artis* (let it be done according to rule)
FLA	fronto-laeva anterior (fetus position)
FLCs	Friend leukemia cells
fld.	*fluidus* (fluid)
flor.	*flores* (flowers)
fl. oz.	*fluidus unica* (fluid ounce)
FLP	fronto-laeva posterior (fetus position)
FLS	follicular lympho-sarcoma
FLT	fronto-laeva transversa (fetus position)
Flu	influenza
f.m.	*fiat mistura* (make a mixture)
Fm	Fermium
FM	frequency modulation
FMC	Free Medical Clinic
FMD	fibro-muscular dysplasia; foot and mouth disease
f.m.d.i.p.	*fiat massa dividenda in pilulae* (let a mass be made and divided into pills)
FME	full mouth extraction
FMEF	forced mid-expiratory flow
FMF	familial Mediterranean fever
FMG	Foreign Medical Graduate
FMN	flavin mono-nucleotide
FMP	first menstrual period
FMS	focal motor seizure
FN	facial nerve; false negative
FNA	fine needle aspiration
FNAB	fine needle aspiration biopsy
FNAC	fine needle aspiration cytology
FNH	focal nodular hyperplasia
FNP	Family Nurse Practitioner
FNT	finger-nose test

FNTC	fine needle transhepatic cholangiography
fo.	*folio* (sheet)
FO	foramen opticum; foramen ovale
FOAM	Fluorouracil, Oncovin, Adriamycin, Mitomycin C
FOAVF	failure of all vital forces
FOB	fecal occult blood; feet on bed; fiber-optic bronchoscopy; foot of bed
FOBS	fiber-optic broncho-scopy
FOD	focus object distance; free of disease
fol.	*folia* (leaves); *folium* (leaf of paper)
FOV	field of vision
f.p.	*fiat potio* (let a potion be made); freezing point
FP	false positive; family planning; family practice; feline pneumonitis; femoral popliteal; flavin phosphate; frozen plasma
FPA	fluoro-phenyl-alanine
FPB	femoral popliteal bypass
FPC	familial polyposis coli; fish protein concentrate
FPG	fasting plasma glucose
FPIA	fluorescence polarization immuno-assay
f. pil.	*fiant pilulae* (let a pill be made)
FPL	flexor pollicis longus
fpm	feet per minute
fps	feet per second
f. pul.	*fiat pulvis* (let a powder be made)
fr.	*frater* (brother)
Fr	father; Francium; French; Friday; from
FR	family report; father; first reaction; fix rate; flocculation reaction; French; Friday; from
FRAT	free radical assay technique (for drugs)
FRC	frozen red cells; functional residual capacity
FRCP	Fellow of the Royal College of Physicians
FRCS	Fellow of the Royal College of Surgeons
FRCVS	Fellow of the Royal College of Veterinary Surgeons
freq.	frequency; frequent
FRFPS	Fellow of the Royal Faculty of Physicians and Surgeons
Fri.	Friday
FRJM	full range of joint movement
FROM	full range of motion
FRP	functional refractory period
FRS	Fellow of the Royal Society
Fru.	fructose

frust.	*frustillatim* (in small pieces)
FRV	functional residual volume
FS	fatigue sign; Fletcher-Suit; flexible sigmoidoscope; flexible sigmoidoscopy; focal spot; full scale
f.s.a.	*fiat secundum artem* (let it be made skillfully)
FSC	Free Standing Clinic
FSD	focal skin distance
FSF	fibrin-stabilizing factor
FSGPA	fetal sulfo-glyco-protein antigen
FSGS	focal and segmental glomerulo-sclerosis
FSH	follicle-stimulating hormone
FSH/LH-RH	follicle-stimulating hormone / luteinizing hormone — releasing hormone
FSH-RF	follicle-stimulating hormone — releasing factor
FSH-RH	follicle-stimulating hormone — releasing hormone
FSI	foam stability index
FSP	fibrin split products; fibrinogen split products
FSR	fusiform skin revision
FSS	flexible sigmoido-scope; flexible sigmoido-scopy
FST	foam stability test
ft.	feet; *fiant* (let there be made); *fiat* (let it be made); foot
FT	family therapy; follow through; full-term; full-time
FT_4	free thyroxine
FTA	fluorescent-absorbed treponemal antibody; fluorescent titer antibody
FTA-AT	fluorescent treponemal antibody absorption test
FTBD	full-term born dead
FTC	Federal Trade Commission
FTG	full thickness graft
FT_3I	free triiodothyronine index
FT_4I	free thyroxine index
ft-lb	foot-pound
FTLB	full-term living birth
FTND	full-term normal delivery
FTR	finger-thumb reflex
FTSG	full thickness skin graft
FTTS	failure-to-thrive syndrome
F/U	follow-up (examination)
FU	Fluoro-uracil; follow-up (examination); fragilitas unguium; fundus uteri
5-FU	5-Fluoro-uracil
FUB	functional uterine bleeding

FUMP	fluoro-uridine mono-phosphate
FUO	fever of undetermined origin; fever of unknown origin
FUT	fibrinogen uptake test
FUTP	fluoro-uridine tri-phosphate
FU-VAC	Fluorouracil, Vinblastine, Adriamycin, Cyclophospha-mide
f.v.	*folio verso* (on the back of the page)
FV	facial vein; femoral vein; fever; fixed value; fluid volume; Friend virus
FVC	forced vital capacity; functional vital capacity
f. ven.	*fiat venaesectio* (let the patient be bled)
FVL	femoral vein ligation
FVR	feline viral rhinotracheitis
FVRT	feline viral rhino-tracheitis
F waves	fibrillation wave; flutter waves
FWB	free weight bearing
fwd	forward (bookkeeping abbreviation)
FWHM	full-width half-maximum
FWR	Felix-Weil reaction
Fx	fracture
Fy	blood group
FYI	for your information
FZ	focal zone
FZS	Fellow of the Zoological Society

~ G ~

γ	Ig = immunoglobulin gamma (abbreviated: immunoglobulin)
γA	IgA = immunoglobulin gamma A (abbr: immunoglobulin A)
γABA	gamma-amino-butyric-acid
γBF	IgBF = immunoglobulin gamma binding factor
γD	IgD = immunoglobulin gamma D (abbr: immunoglobulin D)
γE	IgE = immunoglobulin gamma E (abbr: immunoglobulin E)
γG	IgG = immunoglobulin gamma G (abbr: immunoglobulin G)
γGT	gamma-glutamyl-transferase
γGTp	gamma-glutamyl-trans-peptidase
γM	IgM = immunoglobulin gamma M (abbr: immunoglobulin M)
γR	gamma-ray
GBβHS	group B beta-hemolytic streptococcus
g.	*gravida* (pregnant)
g	gram; gravitation constant; green; ventricular gradient
G	gain; gallop; gamma; gas; gauss; gay; gingival; girl; glass; glossy; glucose; glue; glycerin (glycerine); glycine; good; grade; Greek; guanine; Newtonian constant
G1	histopathologic grade: well differentiated
G2	histopathologic grade: moderately well differentiated
G3	histopathologic grade: poorly differentiated
G4	histopathologic grade: undifferentiated
G_{11}	hexachlophene
Ga	Gallium; gauge
GA	gastric analysis; general anesthesia; general appearance; general assistance; gestational age
G-ABA	gamma-amino-butyric acid
GAD	glutamic acid decarboxylase
GADH	glutamic acid de-hydrogenase

GAG	glycos-amino-glycan
GAGE	gauge
gal.	galactose; gallon
GALSV	gibbon ape lympho-sarcoma virus
GALT	gut-associated lymphoid tissue
GALV	galvanic; gibbon ape lymphosarcoma virus
garg.	*gargarismus* (a gargle)
GAS	general adaptation syndrome
GASA	growth-adjusted sonographic age
GB	gallbladder; Guillain-Barré (syndrome)
GBA	ganglionic blocking agent; gingivo-bucco-axial
GB-BHS	group B beta-hemolytic streptococcus
GBG	glycine-rich B glycoprotein
GBGase	glycine-rich B glycoprotein-ase
GBIA	Guthrie bacterial inhibition assay
GBM	glio-blastoma multiforme; glomerular basement membrane
GBS	gall-bladder series (X-rays); group B streptococcus; Guillain-Barré syndrome
G-c	giga-cycle
GC	ganglion cells; gas chromatography; general closure; gono-coccus; granular casts; guanine cytosine
GCA	giant cell arteritis
g-cal	gram calorie
GCDP	gross cystic disease protein
G-cells	gastrin cells
GC/MS	gas chromatography / mass spectroscopy
GCSA	gross cell surface antigen
G-CSF	granulocyte colony-stimulating factor
GCT	giant cell tumor
Gd	Gadolinium; good
G&D	growth and development
GD	general diagnostics; given dose
GDA	gastro-duodenal artery; germine di-acetate
Gd-DTPA	Gadolinium — diethylene-triamine-penta-acetate
GDM	gestational diabetes mellitus
GDP	guanosine diphosphate
GDS	Geriatric Depression Scale
Ge	Germanium
G/E	granulocyte / erythroid (ratio)
GE	gastro-enterostomy; gastro-esophageal
gel. qu.	*gelatina quavis* (in any kind of jelly)
GEP	gastro-entero-pancreatic

GEPES	gastro-entero-pancreatic endocrine system
GER	German; Germany; gastro-esophageal reflux
GERD	gastro-esophageal reflux disease
GET	gastric emptying time
GET-A	general endo-tracheal anesthesia
GeV	giga electron volt (= 10^9 electron volts = BeV)
GF	gastric fluid; germ-free; gluten-free; growth factor
GFAP	glial fibrillary acidic protein
GFCL	giant follicular cell lymphoma
GFD	gluten-free diet
GFR	glomerular filtration rate
GG	gamma globulin
GGA	general gonadotropic activity
GGE	generalized glandular enlargement
g.g.g.	*gummi guttae gambiae* (gamboge)
GGS	glands, goiter, stiffness
GGT	gamma-glutamyl-transferase
GGTp	gamma-glutamyl-trans-peptidase
GH	growth hormone
GHD	growth hormone deficiency
GH-IF	growth hormone — inhibiting factor
GH-IH	growth hormone — inhibiting hormone
GHPP	Genetically Handicapped Persons Program
GH-RF	growth hormone — releasing factor
GH-RH	growth hormone — releasing hormone
GH-RIH	growth hormone — releasing inhibitory hormone
GHz	giga-Hertz
GI	gastro-intestinal; globulin insulin
GIFT	gamete intra-fallopian transfer
GIK	glucose, insulin, potassium
GIP	gastric inhibitory polypeptide
GIS	gas in stomach; gastro-intestinal system
GIT	gastro-intestinal tract
GITT	glucose-insulin tolerance test
gl.	*glandula* (gland); glass
Gl	Glucinium
g/l	grams per liter (grams per litre)
g/L	grams per liter (grams per litre)
GL	greatest length; glass
GLA	gingivo-linguo-axial
GLC	gas-liquid chromatography
GLC-ECD	gas-liquid chromatography electron capture detector
GLNS	gay lymph node syndrome

GLR	gravity lumbar reduction
glu.	glucose
gluc.	glucose
gm	gram (from French: gramme)
GM	gastric mucosa; Geiger-Mueller
G.M.C.	General Medical Council (British)
GM-CSF	granulocyte-macrophage colony-stimulating factor
GMK	green monkey kidney
GMP	guanosine mono-phosphate
GM-SF	granulocyte-macrophage stimulating factor
G.M.T.	Greenwich Mean Time
GMW	gram-molecular weight
GN	glucose to nitrogen ratio; glomerulo-nephritis; gram-negative
GNB	gram-negative bacteria
GNID	gram-negative intracellular diplococci
GO	general order
GOAT	Galveston Orientation and Amnesia Test
GOP	gynecologic operative procedures
GOT	glutamic-oxaloacetic transaminase
gov't	government
GP	general paresis; general practitioner; gram-positive
G6P	glucose-6-phosphate
GPAIS	guinea pig anti-insulin serum
GPB	gram-positive bacteria
GPC	gastric parietal cell; giant papillary conjunctivitis
GPD	gallons per day; glucose phosphate dehydrogenase
G6PD	glucose-6-phosphate dehydrogenase
GPI	general paralysis of the insane; glucose-phosphate isomerase
GPIMH	guinea pig intestinal mucosal homogenate
GPIPID	guinea pig (intestinal) intra-peritoneal infectious dose
GPKA	guinea pig kidney absorption (test)
GPL	generalized persistent lymphadenopathy
GPM	gallons per minute
GPP	guinea-pig paralysis
GPS	gallons per second; guinea pig serum
GPT	glutamic-pyruvic transaminase
GPTA	graft percutaneous transluminal angioplasty
g.q.	*guttis quibusdam* (with a few drops)
gr.	grain; gravity; green; gross
GR	gastric resection; glutathione reductase (screening)

grad.	*gradatim* (by degrees); gradually; graduate
GRAS	generally recognized as safe
grav.	*gravida* (a pregnant woman; pregnancy)
Grav. 1	first pregnancy
Grav. 2	second pregnancy
Grav. 3	third pregnancy
GRF	gonadotropin releasing factor
GRH	gonadotropin releasing hormone
GRID	gay-related immune disease (deficiency)
GRP	gastrin-releasing peptide
G/S	glucose and saline
GS	general surgery
GSC	gas-solid chromatography
GSD	glycogen storage disease
GSH	Glutathione (Deltathione; Glutathin; Glutinal; Triptide)
GSHV	ground squirrel hepatitis virus
GSN	gray syndrome of the newborn
GSR	galvanic skin response
GSW	gun-shot wound
gt.	*gutta* (drop)
GT	gait training; generation time; glucose tolerance
GT-II	galactosyl transferase — isoenzyme II
GTD	gestational trophoblastic disease
GTF	glucose tolerance factor
GTH	gonado-tropic hormone
GTM	grade, tumor (size and location), metastasis
GTN	gestational trophoblastic neoplasm; glomerulo-tubulo-nephritis; glyceryl tri-nitrate
GTP	guanosine tri-phosphate; glutamyl trans-peptidase
GTRH	gonadotropin releasing hormone
GTS	Gilles de la Tourette's syndrome
gtt.	*guttae* (drops)
GTT	glucose tolerance test
GU	genito-urinary; gastric ulcer; gonococcal urethritis
GUD	genital ulcer disease
GUS	genito-urinary system
gust.	gustation; gustatory
GUSTP	global utilization of streptokinase and tissue plasminogen
gut.	*guttatim* (drop by drop)
GvH	graft versus host
GvHD	graft versus host disease
GvHR	graft versus host reaction

GWI	guinea-worm infection
GX	glycine-xylidide
Gy	gray
Gyn.	gynecologic; gynecological; gynecology; Gynergen (Ergotamine)
GYN	gynecology
gyr.	gyral; gyrate; gyration; gyrectomy; gyrose; gyrospasm; gyrus
GZT	Guilford-Zimmerman Test (of personality)
GZTS	Guilford-Zimmerman Temperament Survey

～ H ～

HAγG	hyperimmune antivariola gamma globulin
HΔV	hepatitis delta virus
HγG	human gamma-globulin
Ⓗ	hypodermic
h.	*hora* (hour)
h	height; Planck's constant (6.626×10^{-34} joule second)
H	enthalpy; *Haemophilus*; halt; hand; head; health; hearing; heat; heavy; height; hemoglobin; hernia; heroin; hip; Hispanic; histamine; history; hole; home; horizontal; hormone; horse; hot; Hounsfield unit; hospital; house; human; husband; hydrate; hydrogen; hydroxyurea; hyper; hypermetropia; hyperopia; hypodermic; hysterectomy; hystrix; physical state of patient; performance state of patient
H-1	Parvovirus
H$^+$	hydrogen ion
^{1}H	hydrogen-1 (protium)
^{2}H	hydrogen-2 (deuterium)
^{3}H	hydrogen-3 (tritium)
H$_2$	histamine-2
H0	normal activity
H1	symptomatic and ambulatory: cares for self
H2	ambulatory: occasionally needs assistance
H3	ambulatory: needs nursing care
H4	bedridden: may need hospitalization
Ha	Hahnium
HA	hallux abductus; head-ache; hem-adsorbent; hemolytic anemia; hepatic artery; hepatitis A; hospital admission; hyaluranic acid; hyper-active
HAA	hepatitis-associated agent; hepatitis-associated antigen
HABF	hepatic artery blood flow
habit.	*habitat* (habit)
HAc	acetic acid
HACE	high-altitude cerebral edema
HACS	hyper-active child syndrome

HAD	Hexamethylmelamine, Adriamycin, DDP
HAE	hepatic artery embolization; hereditary angio-edema
HAFOE	high air flow with oxygen enrichment
HAGG	hyperimmune antivariola gamma globulin
HAHTG	horse anti-human thymus globulin
HAI	hepatic artery infusion
HAM	Hexamethylol-melanine, Adriamycin, Methotrexate; human albumin microspheres; human T-lymphotropic virus type one associated myelopathy
HAMA	human anti-mouse antibody
HAN	hyperplastic alveolar nodules
HANE	hereditary angio-neurotic edema
HAP	heredopathia atactica polyneuritiformis
HAPA	hemagglutinating anti-penicillin antibody
HAPE	high-altitude pulmonary edema
HAPSg	hepatic arterial perfusion scinti-graphy
HAS	hypertensive arterio-sclerosis; hypertensive arterio-sclerotic
HASCVD	hypertensive arterio-sclerotic cardio-vascular disease
HASHD	hypertensive arterio-sclerotic heart disease
HAT	heat and acid test; hypoxanthine-aminopterin-thymidine
haust.	*haustus* (a draft)
HAV	hepatitis A virus
Hb	hemoglobin (haemoglobin)
HB	heart block; hepatitis B
HB_c	hepatitis B core
HB_s	hepatitis B surface
H-2b	mouse cells
HBA	Australian antigen positive hepatitis
HB_cAb	hepatitis B core anti-body
HB_eAb	hepatitis B_e anti-body
HB_sAb	hepatitis B surface anti-body
HBABA	hydroxy-benzene-azo-benzoic acid
HbA,C	hemoglobin A,C (glycohemoglobin)
HBAg	hepatitis B anti-gen
HB_cAg	hepatitis B core anti-gen
HB_eAg	hepatitis B_e anti-gen
HB_sAg	hepatitis B surface anti-gen
HBC	high blood cholestrol
HbCO	carboxy-hemoglobin
HbCV	Haemophilus influenzae type B conjugate vaccine
HBD	hydroxy-butyric dehydrogenase
HbF	fetal hemoglobin

HBF	hepatic blood flow
HbIG	hepatitis B immune globulin
HBIG	hepatitis B immune globulin
HBLV	human B-lymphotropic virus
HBO	hyper-baric oxygenation
HbO_2	oxy-hemoglobin
H_3BO_3	boracic acid; boric acid; orthoboric acid; sassolite
H-bomb	hydrogen bomb
HBP	high blood pressure
HBr	hydro-bromic acid
HbS	hemoglobin — sickle cell
HBS	Hamilton Baldness Scale
Hb-SC	hemoglobin — sickle cell
HBSO	hysterectomy and bilateral salpingo-oophorectomy
HBV	hepatitis B virus
Hc	hematocrit
HC	hair cell; handi-cap; handi-capped; head circumference; head compression; heat capacity; hemi-cystectomy; heparin cofactor; hepatic catalase; hepatitis C; hospital call; hospital consultation; hospital corps; house call; hunger contractions; hunger cure; Hunter's canal; Huntington's chorea; hyaline casts; hyaloid canal; hydro-cortisone
H-CAF	Hexamethylmelamine, Cytoxan, Adriamycin, Fluorouracil
H-CAP	Hexamethylmelamine, Cytoxan, Adriamycin, Platinol
hCC	hepato-cellular carcinoma
HCC	hepato-cellular carcinoma
HCD	heavy chain disease; house call day
HCFA	Health Care Financing Administration
hCG	human chorionic gonadotropin
HCG	human chorionic gonadotropin
HCH	hexachloro-cyclo-hexane
HCHO	formaldehyde
HCl	hydro-chloric acid; hydro-chloride
HCL	hairy cell leukemia
HCM	Health Care Maintenance
HCMV	human cyto-megalo-virus
HCN	house call night; hydro-cya-nic acid; hydrogen cya-nide
HCO_3	bicarbonate
HCP	hereditary copro-porphyria
HCS	hydroxy-cortico-steroids
HCSmt	human chorionic somato-mammo-tropin
HCSUS	HIV cost and services utilization study

Hct	hemato-crit
HCT	hemato-crit; homo-cyto-trophic; human calci-tonin; human chorionic thyrotropin; hydro-chloro-thiazide
HCTz	hydro-chloro-thia-zide
HCV	hepatitis C virus
HCVD	hypertensive cardio-vascular disease
HCW	Health Care Worker
h.d.	*heloma durum* (hard corn); *hora decubitus* (at bedtime)
HD	haemo-dialysis; hard-drive (disk-drive); head; high dosage; hearing deficiency; hearing device; hearing distance; heart disease; hepatitis D; high density; Hodgkin's Disease; hydatid disease
HDC	hanging drop culture
HDCRV	human diploid cell rabies vaccine
HDCV	human diploid cell (rabies) vaccine
HDE	high-dose epinephrine
HDH	heart disease history
HDI	Healthcare Data Interchange
HDLP	high-density lipo-protein
HD-MTX	high-dose methotrexate
HDN	hemolytic disease of the newborn
HDNB	hemolytic disease of the new-born
HDP	hydroxy-dimethyl-pyrimidine
HDRV	human diploid (cell) rabies vaccine
HDS	herniated disk syndrome
HDTV	High Definition Tele-Vision
HDV	hepatitis delta virus; hepatitis D virus
HDVSD	hydrogen detected ventricular septal defect
He	Helium
HE	hemoglobin electrophoresis; hereditary elliptocytosis
HEA	hemorrhage, exudate, aneurysm
HEAL	Health Education Assistance Loan
HEAT	human erythrocyte agglutination test
heb.	*hebdomada* (week)
HEC	hereditary ellipto-cytosis
HEENT	head, eyes, ears, nose, throat
HEK	human embryo kidney; human embryonic kidney
HEL	human embryonic lung
HEOD	Dieldrin
HEP	hemoglobin electro-phoresis
HEPA	high efficiency particulate air (filter)
herb.rec.	*herbarium recentium* (of fresh herbs)
HES	hydroxy-ethyl starch

H&E stain	hematoxylin and eosin stain
HETE	5-hydroxy-eicosa-tetra-enoic (acid)
HETP	hexa-ethyl-tetra-phosphate
Hexa	hexamethylmelamine
Hf	Hafnium
HF	Hageman factor; hair follicle; hay fever; heart failure; heat flow; hemorrhagic fever; hepatic flexure; high flow; high frequency; hydrocele feminae
HFD	high forceps delivery
HFFTTA	hypermobile flat foot with tight tendo Achilles
HFI	hereditary fructose intolerance
HFJV	high-frequency jet ventilation
H-flu	*Haemophilus influenzae*
HFO	high-frequency oscillation
HFP	hexa-fluoro-propylene
HFPPV	high-frequency positive-pressure ventilation
HFS	hemi-facial spasm
HFSH	human follicle-stimulating hormone
HFV	high-frequency ventilation
Hg	hemo-globin; *hydrar-gyrum* (Mercury)
HGA	homo-gentistic acid
hgb.	hemo-globin
hgb-A,C	hemo-globin A and C (glyco-hemoglobin)
hgb-F	hemo-globin — fetal
HGF	hybridoma growth factor; hyperglycemic-glyco-genolytic factor (glucagon)
HGG	human gamma-globulin
hGH	human growth hormone
HGH	human growth hormone
HGHr	human growth hormone recombinant
$Hg(NO_3)_2$	mercuric-nitrate
HGPRT	hypoxanthine-guanine phospho-ribosyl-transfersase
hgt.	height
H&H	hematocrit and hemoglobin
HH	hiatal hernia; hydroxy-hexamide
HHA	hereditary hemolytic anemia
HHB	hemogenic-hemolytic balance
HHD	hypertensive heart disease
HHM	humoral hypercalcaemia of malignancy
HHNKC	hyperosmolar hyperglycemic non-ketotic coma
HHS	health and human services
HHT	hereditary hemorrhage telangiectasia
HHV6	human herpes virus 6

h.i.	*horis intermediis* (at the intermediate hours)
HI	hemagglutination inhibition; high intensity; hydriodic acid
HIA	hemagglutination inhibition antibody
5-HIAA	5-hydroxyl-indole-acetic acid
HIB	*Haemophilus influenzae* type B
HIC	Health Insurance Claim
HID	head, insomnia, depression
HIHA	high-impulsiveness high-anxiety
HILA	high-impulsiveness low-anxiety
HIO₃	iodic acid
HIOMT	hydroxy-indole-o-methyl transferase (acid)
HIP	Health Insurance Plan
HIPC	Health Insurance Plan of California; Health Insurance Purchasing Cooperative
HIPP	Health Insurance Premium Program
HIS	Hospital Information System
hist.	history; histology; histamine; histidine
HIT	hemagglutination inhibition test; hypertrophic infiltrative tendinitis
HIV	human immunodeficiency virus
HIV-Ag	human immune deficiency virus — antigen
HIVIG	hyperimmune intra-venous immuno-globulin
HJ	hepato-jugular
HJR	hepato-jugular reflex
HK	heat-killed; hexo-kinase
HKAFO	hip, knee, ankle, and foot orthosis
HKLM	heat-killed Listeria monocytogenes
H&L	head and leg; head and legs; heart and liver; heart and lung; high and low
HL	half-life; hearing loss; heavy load; histiocytic lymphoma
HLA	human leukocyte antigen; human lymphocyte antigen
HLA-A	human leukocyte antigen — group A
HLA-B	human leukocyte antigen — group B
HLA-C	human leukocyte antigen — group C
HLA-D	human leukocyte antigen — group D
HLA-DR	human leukocyte antigen — group DR
HLA-DR1	human leukocyte antigen — group DR1
HLA-DR5	human leukocyte antigen — group DR5
HLA-L	human leukocyte antigen — group L
hLH	human luteinizing hormone
HLH	human luteinizing hormone

HLHS	hypoplastic left heart syndrome
HLK	heart, liver, kidney
HLP	hairy leuco-plakia; hairy leuko-plakia; hyper-lipo-proteinemia
h.l.s.	*hoc loco situs* (laid in this place)
hLT	human lymphocyte transformation
HLT	human lymphocyte transformation
HLV	herpes-like virus; hypoplastic left ventricle
h.m.	hecto-meter; *heloma molle* (soft corn)
Hm	hyperopia manifest (manifest hyperopia)
HM	hand movement; head movement; heart murmur; high mode; hot milk; human milk; hydatidiform mole
HMA-CMV	human monoclonial antibody — cyto-megalic virus
HMB	homatropine methyl bromide
HMC	heroin, morphine, cocaine
hmct.	hematocrit
HMCT	hematocrit
HMD	hyaline membrane disease
HMG	human menopausal gonadotropin; hydroxy-methyl-glutaryl
HML	human milk lysozyme
HMM	hexa-methyl-melamine
HMO	Health Maintenance Organization; heart minute output
HMP	hexose mono-phosphate; hot moist packs
HMR	histiocytic medullary reticulosis
HMSAS	hypertrophic muscular sub-aortic stenosis
HMSN	hereditary motor and sensor neuropathy
HMSS	hypertrophic muscular subaortic stenosis
HMSst	hypertrophic muscular subaortic stenosis
HMW	high molecular weight
HMW-NCF	high molecular weight — neutrophil chemotactic factor
HMX	heat massage exercise
h.n.	*hoc nocte* (tonight)
H&N	head and neck; head and nose
HN	Head Nurse; hereditary nephritis
HN2	nitrogen mustard (chlormethine; MBA; mechlorethamine)
HNKS	hyperosmolar non-ketotic syndrome
HNO_2	nitrous-acid
HNO_3	nitric-acid
HNP	herniated nucleus pulposus
HNSHA	hereditary non-spherocytic hemolytic anaemia
HNV	has not vomited; has no value
hny.	honey

h/o	history of
Ho	Holmium
H/O	history of
HO	high oxygen
H_2O	water
H_2O_2	hydrogen-peroxide
HOB	head of bed; heat of body
HOCM	hypertrophic obstructive cardio-myopathy
HOH	hard of hearing
HONK	hyper-osmotic non-ketotic (coma)
HOOD	hereditary osteo-onycho-dysplasia
HOP	high oxygen pressure; Hydroxydaunomycin, Oncovin, Prednisone
H_2OsO_4	osmic-acid
hosp.	hospital
HOT	human old tuberculin
Hp	heptoglobin
H+P	history and physical (medical examination)
H&P	history and physical (medical examination)
HP	haemo-perfusion; heat pressure; hemato-porphyrin; high power; high pressure; high protein; horse-power; hot pack; hot packs; house physician; human pituitary
HPA	high-power amplifier; hypothalamo-pituitary-adrenal (axis)
HPAA	hydroxy-phenyl-acetic acid
HpAN	hyperplastic alveolar nodules
HPC	hemangio-peri-cytoma
HPETE	5-hydroxy-peroxy-eicosa-tetra-enoic (acid)
HPF	high-power field
HPFH	hereditary persistence of fetal hemoglobin
HPFSH	human pituitary follicle-stimulating hormone
hPG	human pituitary gonadotropin
HPG	human pituitary gonadotropin
hPL	human placental lactogen
HPL	human placental lactogen
HPLA	hydroxy-phenyl-lactic acid
HPLC	high-performance liquid chromatography; high-pressure liquid chromatography
HPLC-MS	high-performance liquid chromatography mass spectrometry
HPO	high-pressure oxygenation; hypertrophic pulmonary osteoarthropathy
HPO_3	meta-phosphoric-acid

H_3PO_2	hypo-phosphorous-acid
H_2PO_3	phosphorous-acid
H_3PO_4	ortho-phosphoric-acid
$H_4P_2O_6$	hypo-phosphoric-acid
$H_4P_2O_7$	pyro-phosphoric-acid
HPP	hereditary pyro-poikilocytosis; hydroxy-pyrazolo-pymidine
HPRT	hypoxanthine phospho-ribosyl-transferase
HPS	hematoxylin-phyloxine saffron; hypertrophic pyloric stenosis
HPV	Haemophilus Pertussis Vaccine; Human Papilloma Virus
HPVD	hypertensive pulmonary vascular disease
Hpx.	hemopexin
hr	hour
H&R	hysterectomy and radiation
HR	Hartmann Resection; health risk; heart rate; heart reflex; heart replacement; heat rays; heat recovery; hepatic replacement; high rate; high risk; hormone receptor; hospital record; hour
HRA	health risk appraisal; heart rate audiometry
HRBC	horse red blood cells
HRBP	holo-retinol binding protein
HRC	heart-ray cataract; heart-regulating centers
HRF	histamine-releasing factor
HRI	heat rate indicator; height-range indicator
HRIG	human rabies immuno-globulin
hrs.	hours
HRT	heart; hormone replacement therapy
h.s.	*hora somini* (at bedtime)
H&S	hysterectomy and sterilization
HS	half-strength; head surgery; heart sound; heat sensitive; herpes simplex; high school; high sensitivity; homosexual; horse serum; hospital surgery; house staff; house surgeon; Hunter's syndrome; Hurler's syndrome
H_2S	hydrogen-sulfide
HSA	human serum albumin; hypersomnia sleep apnea
HSBI	high serum-bound iron
HSCD	Hand-Schüller-Christian disease
Hse.	hemo-serine
HSE	herpes simplex encephalitis
HSG	herpes simplex genitalis; hystero-salpingo-gram
H_2SiO_3	meta-silisic-acid
H_4SiO_4	ortho-silisic-acid

HSL	herpes simplex labialis
HSM	hepato-splenomegaly
HSMN	hereditary sensory motor neuropathy
H_2SO_3	sulfurous-acid
H_4SO_4	sulfuric-acid
HSR	homogeneously staining region
HSS	hypertrophic subaortic stenosis
HSTS	human-specific thyroid stimulator
HSV	herpes simplex virus
HSV1	herpes simplex virus 1
HSV2	herpes simplex virus 2
HT	heart; heart test; heat; heater; heat tolerance; height; hemagglutination titer; high tension; hot; hyper-tension; hypodermic tablet
HTA	hydroxy-trypt-amine
HTACS	human thyroid adenylate cyclase stimulators
HTC	homozygous typing cells
H-TGL	hepatic tri-glyceride lipase
HTHD	hyper-tensive heart disease
HTLA	human thymus lymphocyte antigen
HTLV	human T-cell leukemia virus
HTLV-I	human T-cell leukemia virus 1
HTLV-II	human T-cell leukemia virus 2
HTLV-III	human T-cell lymphotropic virus 3
htn.	hyper-tension
HTP	hydroxy-trypto-phan
HTR	heater; hemolytic transfusion reaction
hts.	heights
HTS	heat transfer salt
HTSH	human thyroid-stimulating hormone
HTV	herpes-type virus
HU	heat unit; hemagglutinating unit; hydroxy-urea
HuIFN	human inter-feron
h.u.s.	*horae unius spatio* (at the end of one hour)
HUS	hemolytic-uremic syndrome; husband
HuTAS	human thymus anti-serum
HUV	human umbilical vein
H&V	hemigastrectomy and vagotomy
HV	hallux valgus; hallux varus; herpes virus (herpesvirus); high velocity; high voltage; hospital visit
HVA	homo-vanillic-acid
HVD	hypertensive vascular disease

HVE	high-voltage electrophoresis
HVH	herpes virus hominis (herpesvirus hominis)
HVL	half-value layer
HVS	herpes virus simiae (herpesvirus simiae)
hvy.	heavy
HW	hot water
HWB	hot water bottle
HWD	heart-water disease
Hx	hemopexin; hexyl; history
HXIS	Hard X-ray Imaging Spectrometer
Hx/Px	history and physical examination
hypo	hypodermic; hypodermically; sodium-hyposulfite (thiosulfate-sodium)
hyst.	hysterectomy; hysteria; hysterics; hysterorrhexis
hyster.	hysterical; hysterodynia; hysteroepilepsy; hysterogram; hysterography; hysterolysis; hysterometer; hysteropexy; hysteroscope; hysteroscopy; hysterotomy
hystero.	hysterogram; hysterography; hysterometer; hysteroscope; hysteroscopy; hysterotrachelectomy; hysterotracheloplasty; hysterotrachelorrhaphy; hysterotrachelotomy; hysterotraumatism
Hz	Hertz (number of cycles per second)
HZ	herpes zoster (shingles); H zone (Hensen's disk)
HZO	herpes zoster ophthalmicus
HZSIL-TF	herpes zoster specific immune lymphocytic transfer factor
HZV	herpes zoster virus

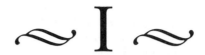

IFNα-2a	interferon alfa — 2a
IFNα-2b	interferon alfa — 2b
IVIγG	intra-venous immune gamma-globulin
I	ampere (electrical current; electrical intensity); in; incision; incisor; India; Indian; injection; inner; inosine; inside; intensity; intercalary; iodine; ion; isotope
^{125}I	radioactive isotope of iodine of atomic weight 125
^{131}I	radioactive isotope of iodine of atomic weight 131
IA	immune adherence; immune associated; index alveolar; infarct anemic; internal auditory; intra-aortic; intra-arterial
IAA	indole-acetic acid
IAB	intra-aortic balloon
IABC	intra-aortic balloon catheter
IABCP	intra-aortic balloon counter-pulsation
IABP	intra-aortic balloon pump; intra-aortic balloon pumping
IAC	internal auditory canal
IACH	idiopathic adrenal cortical hyperplasia
IACPB	intra-aortic counter-pulsation balloon
IADH	inappropriate anti-diuretic hormone
IADHS	inappropriate anti-diuretic hormone syndrome
IADS-AG	intra-arterial digital subtraction angio-graphy
I.A.E.A.	International Atomic Energy Agency
IA-ECG	intra-atrial electro-cardio-gram
IAFI	infantile amaurotic familial idiocy
IAGT	indirect anti-globulin test
IAH	idiopathic adrenal hyperplasia; implantable artificial heart
IAHA	immune adherence hem-agglutination
IAHAA	immune adherence hem-agglutination assay
IAHPS	infection-associated hemo-phagocytic syndrome
IAM	internal auditory meatus
IAP	immunization assistance project; intermittent acute porphyria

IAS	Industrial Applications Society; inter-atrial septum
IASD	inter-atrial septal defect
IASF	intra-amniotic saline infusion
IAT	invasive activity test; iodine-azide test
IAVB	incomplete atrio-ventricular block
IAVD	incomplete atrio-ventricular dissociation
ib.	*ibidem* (in the same place)
IB	immune body; inclusion body
IBB	intestinal brush border
IBC	iron-binding capacity
IBD	inflammatory bowel disease
IBI	intermittent bladder irrigation
IBL	immuno-blastic lymphadenopathy
IBM	inclusion body myositis
IBS	inflammatory bowel syndrome; irritable bowel syndrome
IBV	infectious bronchitis virus
IBW	ideal body weight
i.c.	*inter cibos* (between meals)
IC	immune complex; initial consultation; inspiratory capacity; integrated circuit; intensive care; inter-coolant; inter-costal; intermediate care; intermittent claudication; intermittent count; internal clog; intra-cranial; intra-carotid; intra-cavitary; intra-cellular; intra-cerebral; intra-coronary; intra-cutaneous; irritable colon; ischemic colitis
ICA	ileo-colic artery; internal carotid artery; intra-cranial aneurysm
ICAO	internal carotid artery occlusion
ICC	immune competent cells; Indian childhood cirrhosis; intensive cardiac care; intensive coronary care
ICCE	intra-capsular cataract extraction
ICCMP	idiopathic congestive cardio-myo-pathy
ICCU	intensive cardiac care unit; intensive coronary care unit
ICD	infantile celiac disease; International Classification of Diseases; intra-canthal distance; intrauterine contraceptic device; ischemic cardiac disease; ischemic coronary disease; iso-citrate dehydrogenase; iso-citric dehydrogenase
ICD-9	International Classification of Diseases — 9th revision
ICF	intra-cellular fluid
ICFA	in-complete Freund's adjuvant
ICG	indo-cyanine green

ICH	infantile cortical hyperostosis; intra-cranial hemorrhage
I.C.M.	International Commission for Migration
ICM	immune competence malnutrition; intra-costal margin
I.C.N.	International Council of Nurses
ICNB	inter-costal nerve block
ICP	intra-cranial pressure
ICS	inter-costal space; International College of Surgeons
ICSH	interstitial cell-stimulating hormone
ICT	indirect Coomb's test; inflammation of connective tissue; insulin coma therapy; intermittent cervical traction; insulin clearance test; isovolumic contraction time
ICU	intensive care unit; intensive therapy unit
ICW	intra-cellular water
i.d.	*in dies* (daily)
id.	*idem* (the same)
I&D	incision and drainage
ID	identification; infection droplet; infectious disease; infective dose; internal diameter; intra-dermal
ID$_{50}$	infective dose by 50%; inhibition dose by 50%
IDA	imino-diacetic acid; iron deficiency anemia
id. ac	*idem ac* (the same as)
IDAD	imino-diacetic acid derivatives
IDAGT	in-direct anti-globulin titer
IDAV	immuno-deficiency associated virus
IDD	insulin-dependent diabetes
IDDM	insulin-dependent diabetes mellitus
IDLP	intermediate density lipo-protein
IDM	infant of diabetic mother
IDMS	isotope dilution mass spectrometry
ID/OD	inside diameter / outside diameter (ratio)
IDP	inosine di-phosphate
IDR	intra-dermal reaction
IDS	immunity deficiency state
IDSA	intraoperative digital subtraction angiography
IDTCPP	immuno-deficient thrombo-cyto-penic purpura
IDU	5-iodo-2'deoxy-uridine; idox-uridine
IDV	intermittent demand ventilation
i.e.	*id est* (that is); *injiciatur enema* (let an enema be injected)
I:E	inspiration time : expiration time (ratio)
I/E	inspiration time / expiration time (ratio)
IE	immunizing unit (from German: immunitäts Einheit)

IEEE	Institute of Electrical and Electronics Engineers
IEM	immune electron microscopy; inborn error of metabolism
IEMG	integrated electro-myo-gram
IEOP	immune electro-osmo-phoresis
IEOPh	immune electro-osmo-phoresis
IEP	immuno-electro-phoresis
IEPh	immuno-electro-phoresis
IEPS	invaginate extra-prostatic space
I/f	in full (bookkeeping abbreviation)
IF	immuno-fluorescence; inter-feron; intermittent frequency; internal fluid; intrinsic factor
IFA	immuno-fluorescent antibody; immuno-fluorescent assay; incomplete Freund's adjuvant; indirect fluorescent antibody (test); intrinsic factor antibody
IFCC	International Federation of Clinical Chemistry
IFEP	immuno-fixation electro-phoresis
IFM	internal fetal monitor
Ifn.	interferon
IFN	interferon
IFNA-2a	interferon alfa 2a
IFNA-2b	interferon alfa 2b
IFOS-E	Ifosfamide, Etoposide
IFOS-VP	Ifosfamide, VePesid
IFP	interstitial fluid pressure
IFR	inspiratory flow rate
IFRA	indirect fluorescent rabies antibody (test)
IFT	immuno-fluorescence test
IFV	intracellular fluid volume
Ig	γ = immunoglobulin gamma (abbreviated: immunoglobulin)
IG	immune globulin; intra-gastric
IgA	γA = immunoglobulin gamma A (abbr: immunoglobulin A)
IgBF	γBF = immunoglobulin gamma binding factor
IgD	γD = immunoglobulin gamma D (abbr: immunoglobulin D)
IgE	γE = immunoglobulin gamma E (abbr: immunoglobulin E)
IgG	γG = immunoglobulin gamma G (abbr: immunoglobulin G)
IgM	γM = immunoglobulin gamma M (abbr: immunoglobulin M)
IGT	impaired glucose tolerance

IGV	intrathoracic gas volume
IH	infectious hepatitis; inpatient hospital; insufficiency, hepatic
IHA	indirect hem-agglutination
IHB	incomplete heart block
IHBTD	incomplete hemolytic blood transfusion disease
IHCU	idiopathic hyper-calci-urea
IHD	ischemic heart disease
IHR	index hemo-renal; intrinsic heart rate
IHS	in-house service
IHSA	iodinated human serum albumin
IHSS	idiopathic hypertrophic subaortic stenosis
IH virus	infectious hepatitis virus A
IHW	inner heel wedge
IICP	increased intra-cranial pressure
IIF	indirect immuno-fluorescence
IIFA	indirect immuno-fluorescence antibody
IIP	increased intracranial pressure
IJ	internal jugular
IJC	internal jugular chain
IJP	internal jugular pressure
IJV	internal jugular vein
Il	Illinium
IL	inter-leukin; internal leak; internal lock
I.L.A.	International Leprosy Association
ILBBB	incomplete left bundle branch block
ILD	interstitial lung disorder; ischemic leg disease; ischemic limb disease
ILGF	insulin-like growth factor
ILGF-I	insulin-like growth factor — I
illus.	illustrate; illustrated; illustration
IM	inter-muscular; internal medicine; intra-muscular; intra-muscularly
IMA	inferior mesenteric artery; internal mammary artery
IMAA	iodinated macro-aggregated albumin
IMABP	internal mammary artery by-pass
IMAG	internal mammary artery graft
IMB	inter-menstrual bleeding
IMBC	indirect maximum breathing capacity
IMC	Industrial Medical Council
IMCH	idiopathic myo-cardial hypertrophy
IMCI	inferior myo-cardial infarction
IMF	inferior mesenteric artery; inter-maxillary fixation

IMG	International Medical Graduate
IMH	idiopathic myocardial hypertrophy
IMHT	indirect micro-hemagglutination test
IMI	intra-muscular injection
IMLN	internal mammary lymph node
imm.	immediately; immersion; immune; immunization; immunize
IMN	infectious mono-nucleosis
imp.	imperfect; important; impose; impression; improve; improved
IMP	inosine mono-phosphate
IMPA	incisal mandibular plane angle
impf.	imperfect
IMR	infant mortality rate
IMV	intermittent mandatory ventilation
in.	inch
In	Indium
IN	India; Indian; intra-nasal
INAD	infantile neuro-axonal dystrophy
INAH	iso-nicotinic acid hydrazide
inc.	incorporated; increase; increment
incl.	including
incomp.	incompatibility; incompatible; incompetent
incr	increase; increment
IND	independent; India; Indian; indirect; induced; Investigational New Drug
INEMP	infantile necrotizing encephalo-myelo-pathy
inf.	infant; infected; infection; inferior; infinitive; information; *infra* (below); *infunde* (pour in); *infusum* (infusion)
INFH	ischemic necrosis of femoral head
inflam.	inflammation
INFO	information
INH	iso-nicotinic (acid) hydrazide (Isoniazid; Isonicotinyl)
inhal.	inhalation
init.	initial
inj.	inject; injected; injection; injunction; injury
inj. enem.	*injiciatur enema* (let an enema be injected)
INOP	inter-nuclear ophthalmo-plegia
INPV	intermittent negative pressure ventilation
INR	International Normalized Ratio
ins	insurance (bookkeeping abbreviation)
INS	Immigration and Naturalization Services; insurance
Inst.	install; installation

instil.	instillation
int.	intensive; *intercursus* (intercourse); internal; interval; *intrinsicus* (intrinsic)
interm.	intermediate; intermittent
intermed.	intermediate
interpret.	interpretation
Intl.	international
intox.	intoxicated; intoxication
intsv.	intensive
Io	Ionium
I/O	input and output
I&O	input and output
IO	inferior oblique; intestinal obstruction; intra-ocular
IODSAG	intra-operative digital subtraction angio-graphy
IOI	intra-osseous infusion
IOL	intra-ocular lens
IOML	infra orbito-meatal line
IONP	ischemic optic neuro-pathy
IOP	intra-ocular pressure
IOPD	infectious oral papillomatosis of dogs
IORT	intra-operative radio-therapy
IOTLAP	intra-operative trans-luminal angio-plasty
IP	internal pressure; intra-peritoneal; intra-phalengeal
IPA	Independent Practice Association; iso-propyl alcohol
IPD	inflammatory pelvic disease; inter-pedunculated distance; inter-pupillary distance; intermittent peritoneal dialysis
IPF	idiopathic pulmonary fibrosis
IPG	impedance plethysmography gradient
IPGG	impedance plethysmo-graphy gradient
IPH	idiopathic pulmonary hemosiderosis
IPJ	inter-phalangeal joint
IPK	intractable planter keratosis
IPL	inter-pupillary line
IPM	inches per minute
IPN	infectious pancreatic necrosis
IPOP	immediate post-operative prosthesis
IPP	inflatable penile prosthesis; intermittent positive pressure
IPPA	inspection, percussion, palpation, auscultation
IPPB	intermittent positive pressure breathing
IPPI-O	intermittent positive pressure inflation with oxygen
IPPR	intermittent positive pressure respiration
IPPV	intermittent positive pressure ventilation

IPS	inferior petrosal sinus; infundibular pulmonic stenosis
IPSID	immuno-proliferative small intestinal disease
IPSP	inhibitory post-synaptic potential
IPTG	iso-propyl-thio-galactoside
IPTH	immuno-reactive para-thyroid hormone
i.q.	*idem quod* (the same as)
IQ	intelligence quotient
Ir	Iridium
IR	immune response; inferior rectus; inguinal region; internal radius; internal resistance; internal response
IRA	ileo-rectal anastomosis; immuno-radio-assay
IRAHC	immuno-radio-assayable human chorionic
IRB	Institutional Review Board
IRBBB	incomplete right bundle branch block
IRC	inspiratory reserve capacity
IRDS	idiopathic respiratory distress syndrome
IREM	internal roentgen equivalent, man
IR&F	internal reduction and fixation
IRF	internal reduction and fixation
IRG	immune response genes; immuno-reactive glucagon
IRGH	immuno-reactive growth hormone
IRHGH	immuno-reactive human growth hormone
IRI	immuno-reactive insulin
IRIA	indirect radio-immuno-assay
IRI/G	immuno-reactive insulin / glucose (ratio)
IRMA	immuno-radio-metric assay
IRMVA	intra-retinal micro-vascular abnormalities
IRV	inspiratory reserve volume; inverse ratio ventilation
IS	immune serum; immune suppressor; incentive spirometer; inner surface; intercostal space
ISC	irreversible sickle cell
I.S.C.L.T.	International Society for Clinical Laboratory Technology
I.S.C.V.	International Society for Cardiovascular Surgery
ISDN	iso-sorbide di-nitrate
ISF	internal spermatic fascia; inter-stitial fluid
ISFET	ion-sensitive field-effect transducer
ISG	immune serum globulin
ISH	icteric serum hepatitis
ISIS	International Studies on Infarct Survival
ISK	inter-stitial keratitis
I.S.L.	International Society of Lymphology
ISMA	intrinsic sympatho-mimetic activity
Iso.	isoproterenol

I.S.O.	International Standards Organization
ISS	injury severity score; ion scattering spectroscopy
IST	insulin sensitivity test; insulin shock therapy
I.S.U.	International Society of Urology
ISW	inter-stitial water
IT	inhalation therapy; intensive therapy; intra-tracheal
I.T.A.	International Tuberculosis Association
ITA	internal thoracic artery; intraoperative transluminal angioplasty
ITGT	intra-thoracic glucose tolerance
ITLC	instant thin-layer chromatography
ITLC-SG	instant thin-layer chromatography silica gel
ITP	idiopathic thrombocytopenic purpura; inosine tri-phosphate; intra-thoracic pressure
ITT	insulin tolerance test; internal tibial torsion
IU	immunizing unit; International Unit; intra-uterine
IUCD	intra-uterine contraceptive device
IUD	intra-uterine death; intra-uterine device
IUFB	intra-uterine foreign body
IUFM	intra-uterine fetal malnourished
IUGR	intra-uterine growth rate; intra-uterine growth retardation
IUP	intra-uterine pregnancy
IUT	intra-uterine transfusion
IUU-1	ipsilateral (end-to-end) uretero-ureterostomy — unilateral
IUU-2	ipsilateral (end-to-end) uretero-ureterostomy — bilateral
IV	inter-ventricular; inter-vertebral; intra-vascular; intra-venous (injection); intra-venously; intra-vertebral
IVag	intra-vaginal
IVAP	in vivo adhesive platelet
IVBAT	intra-vascular bronchio-alveolar tumor
IVC	inferior vena cava; inspiratory vital capacity; intra-vascular coagulation
IVCC	intra-vascular consumption coagulation; intra-vascular consumption coagulopathy
IVCCP	intra-vascular consumption coagulo-pathy
IVCD	intra-ventricular conduction defect; intra-ventricular conduction delay
IVCG	inferior vena cava-graphy; intra-venous cholangio-gram; intra-venous cholangio-graphy
IVCP	inferior vena cava pressure

IVD	inter-vertebral disk; intra-venous drug
IVDU	intra-venous drug user
IVF	intra-vascular fluid; in vitro fertilization
IVF-ET	in vitro fertilization embryo transplant
IVGTT	intra-venous glucose tolerance test
IVH	intra-ventricular hemorrhage
IVHA	intra-venous hyper-alimentation
IVIGG	intra-venous immune gamma-globulin
IVJC	inter-vertebral joint complex
IVP	inter-ventricular pressure; intra-venous pyelogram
IVPB	intra-venous piggy-back
IVPG	intra-venous pyelo-gram; intra-venous pyelo-graphy
IVR	idio-ventricular rhythm
IVS	inter-ventricular septum
IVSD	inter-ventricular septal defect
IVSP	inter-ventricular septal perforation
IVT	intra-venous transfusion
IVU	intra-venous urogram; intra-venous urography
IVUG	intra-venous uro-gram; intra-venous uro-graphy
IW	isotopic weight
IWMCI	inferior wall myo-cardial infarction
IWMI	inferior wall myocardial infarction
Ixo.	Ixodes; ixodiasis; ixodic; Ixodidae; ixodin; ixomyelitis

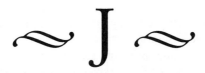

J

J	jail; Japan; Japanese; jaundice; jaw; jerk; jet; Jewish; job; jog; jogging; joint; joule; journal; juice; jump; junior
Ja.	January
JAMA	*Journal of the American Medical Association*
Jan.	January
JBE	Japanese B encephalitis
JBJS	*Journal of Bone and Joint Surgery*
JCA	juvenile chronic arthritis
JCAH	Joint Commission for Accreditation of Hospitals
JCAHO	Joint Commission on the Accreditation of Healthcare Organizations
JCD	Jakob-Creutzfeldt disease
JCI	*Journal of Clinical Investigation*
JCS	Jakob-Creutzfeldt syndrome
jct.	junction
J.D.	*Juris Doctor* (Doctor of Jurisprudence); *Jurum Doctor* (Doctor of Laws)
jej.	jejunum
JEM	*Journal of Experimental Medicine*
JF	joint fluid; joint force; jugular foramen; jugular fossa
JG	jugular ganglion; juxta-glomerular
JGC	juxta-glomerular cell
JGCT	juxta-glomerular cell tumor
JGGI	juxta-glomerular granulation index
JJ	jaw jerk
JKP	jack-knife position (reclining position)
Jl.	July
Jn.	June
JN	Jamaican neuropathy
JNB	jaundice of newborn (*icterus neonatorum*)
JND	just noticeable difference
Jnr.	junior
jnt.	joint
JODM	juvenile onset diabetes mellitus

JP	jugular process; jugular pulse; juxta-position; juxta-pyloric
JPC	junctional premature contraction
JPET	*Journal of Pharmacology and Experimental Therapeutics*
JPS	joint position sense
Jr.	junior
JRA	juvenile rheumatoid arthritis
J.R.C	Junior Red Cross
JS	juxta-spinal; Jarvis' snare; Joffroy's sign
J.S.D.	*Juris Scientiae Doctor* (Doctor of Juristic Science)
jt.	joint
JTC	junctional tachy-cardia
jts.	joints
JTT	Jaeger's test types
JU	Jacob's ulcer
Jul.	July
Jun.	June
juscul.	*jusculum* (soup)
Juv.	juvenile
jux.	*juxta* (near)
JV	jugular vein; jugular venous
JVD	jugular vein distention
JVP	jugular venous pressure; jugular venous pulse
JW	javel water; Javelle water; jaw winking
JXG	juvenile xantho-granuloma
JYF	jungle yellow fever

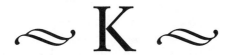

k	Boltzmann's constant; kilo-
K	*kalium* (potassium); Kelvin; kerasin; keratin; keratome; kerosene; kidney; killer; kilometer; kinetic; kinetics; knife; thousand; vitamin K
K^+	kalium ion (potassium ion)
K_a	acid dissociation constant
K_b	base dissociation constant
K_d	dissociation constant
K_e	total exchangeable potassium
K_{eq}	equilibrium constant
K_h	hydrolysis constant
K_i	ionization constant
K_m	Michaelis constant
K_w	water specific constant
K35	Kolman (a urology instrument)
Ka	cathode (from German: kathodos)
KA	keto-acidosis
KAF	conglutinogen activating factor
KAFO	knee-ankle-foot orthosis
KBD	Kashin-Beck disease
KBGS	Kell blood group system
KBr	kalium-bromide (potassium-bromide)
kc	kilo-cycle
Kcal	kilo-calorie
KCC	kathodal closing contraction (cathodal closing contraction)
K-cell	killer cell
KCG	kineto-cardio-gram
kCi	kilo-Curie
KCl	kalium-chloride (potassium-chloride)
$KClO_3$	kalium-chlorate (potassium-chlorate)
KCN	kalium-cyanide (potassium-cyanide)
K_2CO_3	kalium-carbonate (potassium-carbonate)
KCP	knee-chest position

kcps	kilo-cycles per second
KCT	kathodal closure tetanus (cathodal closure tetanus)
KD	kathodal duration (cathodal duration); kissing disease (infectious mononucleosis)
KDA	known drug allergies
KDT	kathodal duration tetanus (cathodal duration tetanus)
keV	kilo-electron-volt
KF	kidney function
KFAB	kidney fixing anti-body
KFF	Kaiser Family Foundation
KFR	Kayser-Fleischer ring
KFS	Klippel-Feil syndrome
kg	kilo-gram
KG	kinder-garten (German: garden of children)
kg.-cal.	kilo-gram-calorie
KGPS	kilo-grams per second
KGS	keto-genic steroid
$KHCO_3$	kalium-bicarbonate (potassium-bicarbonate)
KHD	kinky hair disease; kyphoscoliotic heart disease
KHF	killer helper factor
KHLHC	key-hole limpet hemo-cyanine
kHz	kilo-Hertz
KI	kalium-iodide (potassium-iodide)
KISSC	kidney internal split stent catheter
KIU	kallikrein inhibiting unit
kJ	kilo-joule
KJ	knee jerk
KJR	knee jerk reflex
KK	knee kick; knock-knee
kl	kilo-liter (kilo-litre)
kL	kilo-liter (kilo-litre)
KLS	kidneys, liver, spleen
km	kilo-meter (kilo-metre)
KM	Kanamycin; kilo-meter (kilo-metre)
KMI	Köhler's method of illumination
$KMnO_4$	kalium-permanganate (potassium-permanganate)
kms	kilometers per second (kilometres per second)
KMV	killed measles virus
KMVV	killed measles virus vaccine
kn.	knee; knot; know; knowledge; known
KNO_2	kalium-nitrite (potassium-nitrite)
KNO_3	kalium-nitrate (potassium-nitrate)

KO	knocked out; knock-out
KOC	kathodal opening contraction (cathodal opening contraction)
KOH	kalium-hydroxide (potassium-hydroxide)
koros.	koroscopy
KP	keratitic precipitates; keratitis punctata; kraurosis penis
kPa	kilo-Pascal
KPA	kidney plasminogen activator
KPTT	kaolin partial thromboplastin time
Kr	Krypton
KS	Kallmann's syndrome; Kanner's syndrome; Kaposi's sarcoma; Kaposi's syndrome; Karnofsky scale; keto-steroid; kidney stone; Korsakoff's syndrome
K_2S	kalium-sulfide (potassium-sulfide)
17-KS	17-keto-steroid
KSC	kathodal closing contraction (cathodal closing contraction)
K_2SO_3	kalium-sulfite (potassium-sulfite)
K_2SO_4	kalium-sulfate (potassium-sulfate)
KST	kathodal closing tetanus (cathodal closing tetanus)
KT	Kahn test; Kenny treatment; Krukenberg's tumor
KTM	kata-thermo-meter (cathathermometer)
KUB	kidneys, ureters, bladder (abdominal X-ray)
$K_2U_2O_7$	kalium-uranate (potassium-uranate)
KUS	kidneys, ureters, spleen
kV	kilo-volt
KV	killed vaccine; killed virus; kraurosis vulvae (kraurosis of the vulva)
kVA	kilo-volt-ampere
KVE	Kaposi's varicelliform eruption
KVO	keep vein open
kVp	kilo-volt peak
kW	kilo-watt
KW	kidney worm
kW-hr	kilo-watt per hour
KWI	kidney worm infection
kymo.	kymogram; kymography; kymoscope

~ L ~

Ⓛ	left
l	liter (litre)
L	laboratory; language; late; latex; Latin; lead; leak; leakage; left; leg; lemon; length; lesbian; lethal; leucine; light; lightning; lingual; liter (litre); liver; long; lower; lumbar; lung
L$_+$	limes death
L$_0$	limes zero; lymphatic — no invasion
L1	first lumber vertebrae; lymphatic — superficial invasion
L2	lymphatic — deep invasion; second lumber vertebrae
L3	third lumber vertebrae
l.a.	*lege artis* (according to art)
La	Lanthanum
L&A	light and accommodation (reaction of pupil)
LA	labio-axial; lactic acid; latex agglutination; left anterior; left arm; left atrial; left atrium; left auricle; linguo-axial; local anesthesia; long-acting; lymphocyte activating
LAA	left atrial appendage; leukocyte ascorbic acid
LAAV	lymph-adenopathy associated virus
LAB	laboratory
LABVT	left atrial ball valve thrombus
lac.	lactose
LAC	left atrial contraction; long-arm cast
LAD	lactic acid dehydrogenase; left anterior descending; left axis deviation; leukocyte adhesion deficiency
LAE	left atrial enlargement
laev.	*laevus* (left)
LAF	lymphocyte-activating factor
LAFB	left anterior fascicular block
lag.	*lagena* (flask)
LAG	labio-axio-gingival; lymph-angio-gram
LAH	left atrial hypertrophy
LAHB	left anterior hemi-block
LAI	leukocyte adherence inhibition

LAIA	leukemia-associated inhibitory activity
LAIT	latex agglutination inhibition test
LAK	augmented autologus lymphocytes
LAK cell	lymphokine-activated killer cell
LAL	limulus amebocyte lysate (for measuring endotoxin)
lam	laminectomy; laminotomy
lamin.	laminectomy; laminotomy
lan.	language
LANC	long-arm navicular cast
LAO	left anterior oblique
lap.	laparotomy
LAP	left atrial pressure; leucine amino-peptidase; leukocyte alkaline phosphatase; lyophilized anterior pituitary
LAPAV	lymph-adeno-pathy associated virus
LAPS	lymph-adeno-pathy syndrome
LAR	left arm recumbent; low anterior resection (of rectum)
LAS	left axis shift; lymph-adenopathy syndrome
LASER	Light Amplification by Stimulated Emission of Radiation
LASHB	left anterior superior hemi-block
lat.	lateral
lat. men.	lateral meniscectomy
LATS	long-acting thyroid stimulator
LATSP	long-acting thyroid stimulator protector
LAVH	laparoscopically assisted vaginal hysterectomy
lb.	*libra* (pound)
LB	large bowel; low back; live birth
LBB	left bundle branch
LBBB	left bundle branch block
LBCD	left border of cardiac dullness
LBD	left border dullness
LBF	Lactobacillus bulgaricus factor; liver blood flow
LBGS	Lewis blood group system
LBL	lympho-blastic lymphoma
LBM	lean-body mass
LBO	large bowel obstruction
LBP	low back pain; low blood pressure
LBPP	lower brachial plexus paralysis
lbs.	pounds
LBS	leather bottle stomach (linitis plastica); limy bile syndrome
LBT	louse-borne typhus; lupus band test
LBWI	low birth weight infant

l.c.	*loco citado* (in the place cited)
LC	laparoscopic cholecystectomy; lethal concentration; ligament of Cooper; linguo-cervical; liquid chromatography; low calorie; low concentration
LCA	left circumflex artery; left colic artery; left coronary artery; leukocyte common antigen
LCAT	lecithin cholesterol acyl-transferase
LCCS	low cervical cesarean section
LCD	Liquid Crystal Display; liquor carbonis detergens; lobster-claw deformity
LCFA	long-chain fatty acid
LCG	liquid chromato-graphy
LCIS	lobular carcinoma in-situ
LCL	large cell leukemia; lympho-cytic leukemia
LCLS	lympho-cytic lympho-sarcoma
LCM	left costal margin; lymphatic chorio-meningitis
LCP	Legg-Calvé-Perthes (disease)
LCS	lateral cerebral sulcus
LCTG	liquid crystal thermo-gram; long-chain tri-glyceride
LCWI	left cardiac work index
l.d.	*loco dolenti* (to the painful spot)
LD	large dose; learning defect; learning disorder; learning disturbance; Leber's disease; left deltoid; Legionnaires' disease; lethal dose; lie detector; light difference; limited dose; liquid diet; Little's disease (cerebral palsy); loco disease; low dose; Lyme disease
LD_{50}	lethal dose — 50% (median)
LD_{100}	lethal dose — 100% (invariable)
LDA	left descending artery; left dorso-anterior
LDCC	lectin-dependent cellular cytoxicity
LDH	lactate de-hydrogenase; lactic de-hydrogenase
LDHG	lactate de-hydro-genase; lactic de-hydro-genase
LDHG virus	lactic de-hydro-genase virus
LDLP	low-density lipo-protein
LDLPC	low-density lipo-protein cholesterol
LDP	left dorso-posterior (fetus position)
LDR	labor, delivery, recovery
L.D.S.	Licentiate in Dental Surgery
LDUB	long double upright brace
LDV	lateral distant view
LE	left eye; lower extremity; lupus erythematosus
LEA	lower extremity amputation

127

LE cell	lupus erythematosus cell
LED	light-emitting diode; lupus erythematosus disease; lupus erythematosus disseminatus
LE factor	lupus erythematosus factor
LEOPARD	Lentigines, Electrocardiographic abnormalities, Ocular hypertelorism, Pulmonary stenosis, Abnormalities of genitalia, Retardation of growth, sensori-neural Deafness
LEOS	Lasers and Electro-Optics Society
LE prep.	lupus erythematosus (cell) preparation
LES	local excitatory state; lower esophageal sphincter
LESP	lower esophageal sphincter pressure
LE test	lupus erythematosus (cell) test
leu.	leucine
lev.	*levis* (light)
LF	Lassa fever; lenticular fossa; limit flocculation; lipotropic factors; liver failure; liver flap (asterixis); liver function; lower left; low fat; low forceps; low frequency
LFA	left femoral artery; left fore-arm; left fronto-anterior (fetus position)
LFAP	low friction arthro-plasty
LFD	lactose-free diet; least fatal dose; low-fat diet; low forceps delivery
LFO	limbus fossa ovalis
LFP	left fronto-posterior (fetus position)
LFPPV	low-frequency positive-pressure ventilation
LFT	latex flocculation test; left fronto-transverse (fetus position); liver function test
LG	labial glands; lacrimal gland; large; left gluteal; linguo-gingival; Littré's glands (urethral glands); lympho-graphy
LGA	large for gestational age
LGB	low grade bleeding; Landry-Guillain-Barré (syndrome)
LGF	low grade fever
LGH	lacto-genic hormone
LGL	Lown-Ganong-Levine (syndrome); large granular lymphocyte
LGN	lateral geniculate nucleus; lobular glomerulo-nephritis
LGS	Lennox-Gastut syndrome
LGT	low grade temperature
lgth.	length
LGV	lympho-granuloma venereum
LH	left hand; left heart; low heat; luteinizing hormone

LHF	left heart failure
LHFSH	luteinizing hormone follicle-stimulating hormone
LHL	left hepatic lobe
LHRF	luteinizing hormone-releasing factor
LHS	left hand side
LHT	left hyper-tropia; light
Li	Lithium
LI	linguo-incisal; labelling index (labeling index)
LIAFI	late infantile amaurotic familiar idiocy
lib.	liberal; libidinous; libido; library
LIBC	latent iron-binding capacity
LiBr	lithium-bromide
LIBS	Lendrum's inclusion-body stain
LICM	left inter-costal margin
Li_2CO_3	lithium-carbonate
LICS	left inter-costal space
LIF	left iliac fossa; leukocyte inhibitory factor
LIFO	Last In, First Out
LIFT	lymphocyte immuno-fluorescent test
lig.	ligament; ligamenta; ligementum
LIH	left inguinal hernia
LIHR	laparoscopic inguinal hernia repair
LIMA	left internal mammary artery
Lin. ac.	linear acceleration; linear accelerator
LINAC	linear acceleration; linear accelerator
Li_2O	lithium-oxide
LiOH	lithium-hydroxide
liq.	liquid; *liquor* (a liquor; liquid)
LIR	left iliac region
LIS	left intercostal space; lobular in-situ
LIVIM	lethal intestinal virus of infant mice
LK	left kidney; left knee
Lkc.	leukocyte
LKP	lamellar kerato-plasty
LKS	liver, kidneys, spleen
LL	large lymphocyte; left leg; left lower; left lung; lower lobe
LLB	long-leg brace
LLC	liquid-liquid chromatography; long-leg cast
LLCG	liquid-liquid chromato-graphy
LLE	left lower extremity
LLF	Laki-Lorand factor
LLL	left lower leg; left lower lobe; left lower lung

LLQ	left lower quadrant
LLR	left lumbar region
LLRP	left lateral recumbent position
LLS	lazy leukocyte syndrome; long-leg splint
lm.	lumen
LM	linguo-mesial
LM427	Ansamycin
LMA	left mento-anterior (fetus position)
LMCA	left main coronary artery; left middle cerebral artery
LMF	leukocyte mitogenic factor
LML	left medial lateral; left middle lobe
LMM	lentigo maligna melanoma
LMN	lower motor neuron
LMND	lower motor neuron disease
LMP	last menstrual period; left mento-posterior (fetus position)
LMT	left mento-transverse (fetus position)
LMWD	low molecular weight dextran
LMWH	low molecular weight heparin
LN	lipoid nephrosis; lupus nephritis; lymph node
LNG	liquefied natural gas
LNMP	last normal menstrual period
LNPF	lymph node permeability factor
LO	libidinal object (love object); linguo-occlusal
LOA	leave of absence; left occipito-anterior (fetus position); level of activities; level of activity
LOB	loss of blood; loss of brain; loss of bone
LOC	laxative of choice; level of consciousness; local; locate; location; loss of consciousness
LOCS	lens opacities classification system
LOD	lack of data
log.	logarithm
LOL	left occipito-lateral (fetus position)
LOM	lack of medicine; left otitis media; loss of motion
LOP	left occipito-posterior (fetus position)
LOPP	Leukeran, Oncovin, Procarbazine, Prednisone
LOQ	lower outer quadrant
LOR	law of refreshment
LOS	length of stay; length of surgery
lot.	*lotio* (lotion)
LOT	left occipito-transverse (fetus position)
LOW	low on water

L/P	lactate / pyruvate (ratio)
LP	latency period; light perception; lightning pain; lipo-protein; low power; low pressure; low protein; lumbar puncture; lymphoid plasma
LPA	latex partial agglutination; left pulmonary artery
LPC	lead pipe contraction
LPD	low protein diet
l.p.f.	low-power field (microscope)
LPF	leukocytosis-promoting factor; low-pressure fluid; lymphocytosis-promoting factor
LPFB	left posterior fascicular block
LPG	liquefied propane gas
LPH	lipotropic hormone; lipotropin
LPHB	left posterior hemi-block
LPL	lipo-protein lipase
l.p.m.	liters per minute (litres per minute)
LPN	Licensed Practical Nurse
LPO	left posterior oblique (fetus position)
LPOCA	Leucogen, Prednisone, Oncovin, Cytarabine, Adriamycin
LPS	lead-pencil stools; lipo-poly-saccharide
LPV	left pulmonary vein
LQ	lower quadrant
Lr	Lawrencium
L→R	left to right; move from left to right
L&R	left and right
LR	labor room; lateral rectus; laughter reflex; light reaction; light reflex; light-resistant; lower right
LRA	low rectal anastomosis
L.R.C.P.	Licentiate of the Royal College of Physicians
L.R.C.S.	Licentiate of the Royal College of Surgeons
LRD	local regional disease
L.R.F.P.S.	Licentiate of the Royal Faculty of Physicians and Surgeons
LRH	luteinizing-releasing hormone
LRI	lacted Ringer's injection; lower respiratory illness
LRM	left radical mastectomy
LRQ	lower right quadrant
LRS	lactated Ringer's solution
LRT	lower respiratory tract
L:S	lecithin : sphingomyelin (ratio)
L/S	lecithin / sphingomyelin (ratio)
L.S.	*locus sigilli* (place of the seal; place of the signature)

LS	left side; leg surgery; love-sick; lumbo-sacral; lympho-sacral
LSA	left sacro-anterior (fetus position)
LSB	left scapular border; left sternal border
LScA	left scapulo-anterior (fetus position)
LSCG	liquid-solid chromato-graphy
LScP	left scapulo-posterior (fetus position)
LSCS	lower segment cesarean section
LSCV	left sub-clavian vein
LSD	least significant digit; lipid storage disease; low-salt diet; lumpy skin disease (virus); lysergic acid diethylamide
LSF	low saturated fat (diet)
LSH	lutein-stimulating hormone; lymphocyte-stimulating hormone
LSI	large-scale integration
LSK	liver, spleen, kidneys
LSL	left sacro-lateral (fetus position)
LSM	late systolic murmur
LSO	lumbo-sacral orthosis
LSP	left sacro-posterior (fetus position)
LSS	life-saving service; life-saving station; life-support system; low-salt syndrome; lumbo-sacral spine
LST	last simple trial; left sacro-transverse (fetus position); light sense tester
LT	left thigh; left turn; leuko-triene; levo-thyroxine; ligament of Treitz; light; low tension; lung transplantation; lympho-toxin
LTA	lipo-teichoic acid
LTB	laryngo-tracheo-bronchitis
LTB$_4$	leuko-triene B$_4$
LTC	long-term care
LTC$_4$	leuko-triene C$_4$
LTCF	long-term-care facility
ltd.	limited
LTD	limited; long-term diagnosis
LTF	lymphocyte-transforming factor
LTH	luteo-tropic hormone (prolactin)
LTM	laryngo-tracheo-malacia; long-term memory
LTP	long-term prognosis
LTR	letter; lighter; long terminal repeat
LTS	laryngo-tracheal stenosis; long-term survival

LTT	lymphocyte transformation test
Lu	Lutetium
L&U	left and upper
LU	large unit; left upper; ligature of ureter
LUE	left upper extremity
Lues I	primary syphilis
Lues II	secondary syphilis
Lues III	tertiary syphilis
LUL	left upper limb; left upper lobe; left upper lung
LUQ	left upper quadrant
LURF	luteinized un-ruptured follicle
LV	leave; left ventricle; leukemia virus; leukopheresis vulvae; live virus; live; low viscosity; low voltage; lues venerea (syphilis); lumbar vertebra; lupus vulgaris
LVAD	left ventricular assist device
LVB	Lomustine, Vinblastine, Bleomycin
LVD	left ventricular dysfunction
LVDP	left ventricular diastolic pressure
LVDV	left ventricular diastolic volume
LVE	left upper extremity; left ventricular ejection; left ventricular enlargement
LVEDP	left ventricular end-diastolic (transmural) pressure
LVEDV	left ventricular end-diastolic volume
LVEF	left ventricular ejection fraction
LVESV	left ventricular end-systolic volume
LVET	left ventricular ejection time
LVF	left ventricular failure; low-voltage foci
LVH	left ventricular hypertrophy
LVHT	left ventricular hyper-trophy
LVN	Licensed Visiting Nurse; Licensed Vocational Nurse
LVP	left ventricular pressure; lysine vaso-pressin
LVPP/LVET	left ventricular preejection period / left ventricular ejection time
LVR	Leucovorin (Citrovorum factor)
LVS	left ventricular strain
LVSP	left ventricular systolic pressure
LVSV	left ventricular stroke volume
LVSW	left ventricular stroke work
LVSWI	left ventricular stroke work index
LVTP	left ventricular transmular pressure
LVW	left ventricular wall; left ventricular width
L&W	living and well

LW	low water
LWM	Lee-White method
lx.	lux
lymphs.	lymphocytes
lys.	lysin; lysine; lyssoid
lyso.	lysolecithin
lyx.	lyxose
LZ	ligament of Zinn

～ M ～

μ	letter m in Greek; mass absorption coefficient; micro-; micron; population mean; the heavy chain of IgM
μA	micro-ampere
μc	micro-calorie; calorie
μC	micro-Coulomb
μCi	micro-Curie
μEq.	micro-equivalent
μF	micro-Farad
μg	micro-gram
μI	micro-ampere
μl	micro-liter (micro-litre)
μL	micro-liter (micro-litre)
μm	micro-meter (micro-metre)
μM	micro-molar
μmg	micro-milli-gram
μmm	micro-milli-meter (micro-milli-metre)
μP	micro-processor
μR	micro-Roentgen
μs	micro-second
μsec	micro-second
μU	micro-unit
μV	micro-volt
μW	micro-watt
μμCi	micro-micro-Curie (pico-Curie)
μμg	micro-micro-gram (pico-gram)
mμ	milli-micron
MSαFP	maternal serum alpha-feto-protein
Ⓜ	murmur
m.	mass; median; meter (metre); milli-; *misce* (mix); *mistura* (mixture); *musculus* (muscle)
M	macerate; magnetic; main; major; male; man; manual; married; marrow; mass; maximum; maximal; meaning; measurement; medication; medicine; medium; meeting; mega-; Megestrol; men; mesial; metastasis; meter

	(metre); Methionine; Mexican; Mexico; mice; middle; mile; milk; minimum; minimal; minor; minute; mistake; Mitomycin; mitotic; mix; mixture; molar; mole; Monday; monkey; month; morning; mother; mouse; mouth; mucoid; multiply; multiple; murmur; muscle; music; mute; myopia
m^2	square meter (square metre)
M_1	mitral valve closure — first sound
M_2	mitral valve closure — second sound
M0	tumor with no distant metastasis
M1	tumor with distant metastasis
M_L	left electrode
M_R	right electrode
mA	milli-ampere
Ma	March; Masurium (Technetium)
M.A.	*Magister Artium* (Master of Arts)
MA	mandelic acid; mean arterial; Medic Alert; Mediterranean anemia (Thalassemia); menstrual age; mental age
MAA	macro-aggregated albumin; melanoma-associated antigen
MABOP	Mechlorethamine, Adriamycin, Bleomycin, Oncovin, Prednisone
MABP	mean arterial blood pressure
mac.	*macerare* (macerate)
MAC	maximum allowable concentration; membrane attack complex; Methotrexate, Adriamycin, Cytoxan; *Mycobacterium avium* complex
MACC	Methotrexate, Adriamycin, Cyclophosphamide, CCNU
MACI	membrane attack complex inhibitor
MACOP-B	Methotrexate, Adriamycin, Cytoxan, Oncovin, Prednisone, Bleomycin
M.A.C.P.	Master of the American College of Physicians
MACS	Multicenter AIDS Cohort Study
MAD	maximal acid output
MAE	move all extremities
MAF	macrophage activation factor; macrophage agglutination factor
mag.	magnification; magnify; magnitude; *magnus* (large)
MAgF	macrophage agglutination factor
MAHA	micro-angiopathic hemolytic aneurysm
MAI	*Mycobacterium avium* intracellularis
MAIC	maximum allowable ingredient concentration
MAL	mid-axillary line

malig.	malignant
mam.	*mamma* (breast); *mammosus* (mammose)
MAM	methyl-azo-methanol
man.	manikin; manipulation; *manipulus* (a handful); manual; manus
manip.	manipulation; *manipulus* (handful)
MAO	maximum acid output; mono-amine oxidase
MAOI	mono-amine oxidase inhibitor
MAP	mean aortic pressure; mean arterial pressure; megaloblastic anemia of pregnancy; methy-acetoxy-progestrone; muscle-action potential
MAPF	micro-atomized protein food
Mar.	March; margin; marginal; margination
MAS	meconium aspiration syndrome; milk-alkali syndrome; movement alarm signal
MASER	Microwave Amplification by Stimulated Emission of Radiation; Molecular Application by Stimulated Emission of Radiation
MASH	Mobile Army Surgical Unit
mass.	*massa* (mass)
mast.	mastalgia; mastication; masturbation
MAST	medical anti-shock trousers; Michigan Alcohol Screening Test; military anti-shock treatment; military anti-shock trousers
MAT	Miller-Abbott tube
MATB	*Mycobacterium avium* tuberculosis
matut.	*matutinus* (in the morning)
MAVIS	mobile artery and vein imaging system
max.	maxillary; *maximus* (maximum)
m.b.	*misce bene* (mix well)
Mb	myoglobin
M.B.	*Medicinae Baccalaureus* (Bachelor of Medicine)
MB	main block; mega-byte; mesio-buccal; methylene blue
M.B.A.	Master of Business Administration
MBA	Mechlorethamine (Nitrogen mustard; HN2); methyl-bovine albumin
M-BACOD	Methotrexate, Bleomycin, Adriamycin, Cytoxan, Oncovin, Dexamethasone
MBAP	megalo-blastic anemia of pregnancy
MBC	maximum breathing capacity; Methotrexate, Bleomycin, Cisplatin; minimal bactericidal concentration
MBD	Methotrexate, Bleomycin, DDP; methylene blue dye; minimal brain damage; minimal brain dysfunction

MBDS	minimal brain dysfunction syndrome
MBF	mean blood flow
MBK	methyl-butyl-ketone
MBL	menstrual blood loss; minimal bactericidal level
MBO	mesio-bucco-occlusal
MBP	mean blood pressure; melitensis, bovine, porcine; mesio-bucco-pulpal; Methotrexate, Bleomycin, Platinol; myelin basic protein
MBSA	methylated bovine serum albumin
mc	milli-Curie
mC	milli-Coulomb
Mc	mega-cycle
M+C	morphine and cocaine
M&C	morphine and cocaine
M.C.	*Magister Chirurgiae* (Master of Surgery); Medical Corps
MC	major cut; mast cell; mature cataract; maximum concentration; medical case; mega-Curie; mero-cyanine; meta-carpal; mineralo-corticoid; minor cut; myo-carditis; Mitomycin C
MCA	Megestrol, Cytoxan, Adriamycin; mid-colic artery; middle cerebral artery; multiple congenital anomaly
MCAB	mono-clonial anti-body
MCAT	Medical College Admission Test
MCB	myo-cardial band
MCBF	myo-cardial blood flow
MCBR	minimum concentration of bili-rubin
MCCF	myo-cardial contractile force
MCCNU	methy-CCNU (MeCCNU; Semustine)
MCCU	mobile coronary care unit
MCD	mean cell diameter; mean corpuscular diameter; medullary cystic disease; myo-cardial disease
MCDF	myo-cardial depressant factor
MCF	macrophage chemotactic factor; malignant catarrhal fever; Mitoxantrone, Cytoxan, Fluorouracil; myo-cardial fibrosis
MCF-A	malignant catarrhal fever — African
mcg	micro-gram
MCGF	most cell growth factor
M.Ch.	*Magister Chirurgiae* (Master of Surgery)
MCH	mean corpuscular hemoglobin; medical case history
MCHA	muscle-contraction head-ache
MCHC	mean corpuscular hemoglobin concentration

MCHg	mean corpuscular hemo-globin
MCHgC	mean corpuscular hemo-globin concentration
mCi	milli-Curie
MCi	mega-Curie
MCI	mean cardiac index; myo-cardial infarction
mCid	milli-Curie-day
mCih	milli-Curie-hour
MCL	medial collateral ligament; mid-clavicular line; mid-costal line; most comfortable loudness
MCLD	meta-chromatic leuko-dystrophy
MCM	major cross match
MCP	Melphalan, Cytoxan, Prednisone; meta-carpo-phalangeal
MCPB	membranous cyto-plasmic body
MCPJ	meta-carpo-phalangeal joint
Mc.p.s.	mega-cycles per second
MCR	metabolic clearance rate
MCR-S	metabolic clearance rate of steroid
M-CSF	macrophage colony-stimulating factor
MCT	mean circulation time; mean corpuscular thickness; medullary carcinoma of thyroid
M-CT-CG	metrizamide computed tomography cisterno-gram; metrizamide computed tomography cisternography
MCTD	mixed connective tissue disease
MCTG	medium-chain tri-glyceride
MCTS	Medi-Cal transaction software
MCV	mean corpuscular volume
m.d.	*more dicto* (as directed)
Md	Mendelevium
M.D.	*Medicinae Doctor* (Doctor of Medicine)
MD	maximum dose; McArdle's disease; medical doctor; Ménière's disease; mental deficiency; mentally deficient; mesio-distal; minimum dose; muscular dystrophy; myocardial damage; myocardial disease; mini-disc
MDA	mento-dextra anterior (fetus position); 3,4-methylene-dioxy-amphetamine; minimum detectable activity
MDAC	multiple dose-activated charcoal
MDC	minimum detectable concentration
MDF	multiple daily fractionation; myocardial depressant factor
MDHG	maleate de-hydro-genase
MDI	manic-depressive illness; multiple daily injection

MDM	mid-diastolic murmur
mdnt.	mid-night
MDP	major duodenal papilla; manic-depressive psychosis; mento-dextra posterior (fetus position); muramyl-di-peptide
MDR	manic-depressive reaction; minimum daily requirement; multi-drug resistance
MDRTB	multi-drug resistant tuberculosis
M.D.S.	Master of Dental Surgery
MDS	myelo-dyplastic syndrome
MDT	mento-dextra transverse (fetus position)
MDUO	myocardial disease of unknown origin
MDY	month, date, year
Me	methyl
M:E	myeloid cell : erythroid cell (ratio)
M/E	myeloid cell / erythroid cell (ratio)
ME	macular edema; Medical Examiner; middle ear
2-ME	2-mercapto-ethanol
MEA	mercapto-ethyl-amine; multiple endocrine abnormalities
MEAP	multiple endocrine adeno-pathy
MECC	multiplicative expanding cell compartment
MeCCNU	methyl-CCNU (MCCNU; Semustine)
med.	median; medical; *medicamentum* (medicine)
MED	minimal effective dose; minimal erythema dose
MEDAC	Multiple Endocrine Deficiency Autoimmune Candidiasis
MEDLARS	Medical Literature and Retrieval System
MEDLINE	MEDLARS' on-line segment
MEF	maximum expiratory flow
MEFR	maximum expiratory flow rate
MEFV	maximum expiratory flow volume
MEG	magneto-encephalo-gram; magneto-encephalo-graphy
mega-	one million
MEGX	mono-ethyl-glycine-xylidide
MEK	methyl-ethyl-ketone
MEL	mouse erythro-leukemia; murine erythro-leukemia
MELASE	Mitochondrial Encephalopathy Lactic Acidosis and Stroke-like Episode
MEM	macrophage electrophoretic mobility (test); memory
MEMS	Medical Event Monitoring System
m.e.n.	*mane et nocte* (morning and night)
MEN	multiple endocrine neoplasia
MEN-1	multiple endocrine neoplasia type 1

MEN-2	multiple endocrine neoplasia type 2
MEN-3	multiple endocrine neoplasia type 3
MEP	motor-evoked potential
MEPP	miniature end-plate potential
mEq	milli-equivalent
mEq/l	milli-equivalent per liter (milli-equivalent per litre)
mEq/L	milli-equivalent per liter (milli-equivalent per litre)
MER	mean ejection rate; methanol extraction residue
m.e.s.	*misce et signa* (mix and write)
MET	metabolic equivalent of task
META	micro-encapusulated tumor assay
mets.	metastasis
meV	milli-electron volt
MeV	mega-electron volt (million electron volts)
MEV	mega-electron volt (million electron volts)
m.f.	*mistura fiat* (let a mixture be made)
mF	milli-Farad
MF	macula flava; Malta fever; Mediterranean fever (brucellosis); medium frequency; micro-Farad; microscopic factor; Mitomycin, Fluorouracil; mycosis fungoides
MFAT	multi-focal atrial tachycardia
MFATc	multi-focal atrial tachy-cardia
MFCG	Mycosis Fungoides Cooperative Group
MFD	mid-forceps delivery; minimum fatal dose
mfg.	manufacturing
MFGDA	milk-fat globule-derived antigen
MFH	malignant fibrous histiocytoma
MFHC	malignant fibrous histio-cytoma
MFP	mono-fluoro-phosphate
MFR	mucus flow rate
MF-SS	mycosis fungoides Sézary syndrome
MFT	muscle function test
mg	milli-gram
mg%	milli-grams percentage
Mg	Magnesium
MG	main gate; main group; Marcus Gunn (pupil); Mecklel's ganglion; mesio-gingival; methyl glucoside; muscle group; myasthenia gravis
mg/cc	milli-grams per cubic centimeter
$MgCl_2$	magnesium-chloride
mg/dl	milli-grams per deci-liter (milli-grams per deci-litre)
mg/dL	milli-grams per deci-liter (milli-grams per deci-litre)

mg/h	milli-grams per hour
mgh	milli-gram-hour
mg/kg	milli-grams per kilo-gram
mg/l	milli-grams per liter (milli-grams per litre)
mg/L	milli-grams per liter (milli-grams per litre)
mgm	milli-gram
mgmt.	management
MGN	membranous glomerulo-nephritis
MgO	magnesium-oxide
mgr.	manager
MGSA	melanoma growth stimulating activity
MgSO$_3$	magnesium-sulfite
MgSO$_4$	magnesium-sulfate
mgt.	management
mgtis.	meningitis
mgtt.	micro-guttae (micro-drop); mini-guttae (mini-drop)
MGUS	Monoclonal Gammopathy of Undetermined Significance; Monoclonal Gammopathy of Unknown Significance
mH	milli-Henry
MH	menstrual history; mental health
MHA	micro-hem-agglutination; mixed hem-adsorption
MHAA-TP	micro-hem-agglutination assay for Treponema pallidum
MHC	Mexican hat cell (target cell)
MHCC	major histo-compatibility complex
MHD	mean hemolytic dose; minimum hemolytic dose
MHMA	methoxy-hydroxy-mandelic acid
MHN	massive hepatic necrosis
MHPG	methoxy-hydroxy-phenyl-glycol
MHR	maximal heart rate
MHVD	Marek's herpes virus disease
MHW	medial heel wedge
MHz	mega-Hertz
mi.	mile
MI	maturation index; mental illness; mercapto-imidazole; mesenteric ischemia; mitotic index; mitral insufficiency
MIA	missing in action
MIBG	meta-iodo-benzl-guanidine
MIBK	methyl-iso-butyl-ketone
MIC	Maternal and Infant Care; microbe; microphone; microscope; minimal isorrheic concentration; minimum inhibitory concentration

MICU	Medical Intensive Care Unit
MID	mesio-inciso-distal; middle; minimum infective dose; minimum inhibiting dose; multi-infarct dementia
MIF	micro-immuno-fluorescence; microphage inhibitory factor; migration inhibitory factor; mixed-immuno-fluorescence; Müllerian inhibitory factor
MIFR	maximum inspiratory flow rate
mil.	milli-liter (milli-litre)
min.	mineral; *minimum* (minim); minor; minute
mins.	minutes
MIO	minimal identifiable odor
MIP	maximum inspiratory pressure
MIPS	Myocardial Isotope Perfusion Scan
MIRD	Medical Internal Radiation Dose
MIRI	Myocardial Infarction Recovery Index
MIS	Müllerian inhibiting substance
misc.	miscarriage; miscegenation; miscellaneous
mist.	mistake; *mistura* (mixture)
mit.	*mitte* (send)
MIT	mono-iodo-tyrosine
Mito-C	Mitomycin C
mitt.	*mitte* (send)
mit. x tal.	*mitte decam tales* (send 10 like this)
mIU	milli-International Unit
mixt.	mixture
mJ	milli-Joule
MJ	mari-juana
MJS	medial joint space
mk	mark
MK	monkey kidney; Munro Kern (maneuver)
MKC-CSA	mega-karyo-cytic colony-stimulating activity
mks	marks; meter-kilogram-second
ml.	milli-liter (milli-litre)
mL	milli-liter (milli-litre)
M:L	monocyte : lymphocyte (ratio)
M/L	monocyte / lymphocyte (ratio)
ML	mesio-lingual; mid-line; middle lobe; muco-lipidosis
ML1	muco-lipidosis type 1
ML2	muco-lipidosis type 2
ML3	muco-lipidosis type 3
ML4	muco-lipidosis type 4
MLA	mento-laeva anterior (fetus position); monocytic

	leukemia acute
MLB	monaural loudness balance
MLC	minimum lethal concentration; mixed leukocyte culture; mixed lymphocyte culture
MLD	manual lymph drainage; median lethal dose; minimum lethal dose
MLHc	malignant lymphoma histio-cytic
MLI	mesio-linguo-incisal
MLNS	Mucocutaneous Lymph Node Syndrome
MLO	mesio-linguo-occlusal
MLP	mento-laeva posterior (fetus position); mesio-linguo-pulpal
MLR	mixed lymphocyte reaction
MLT	mento-laeva transverse (fetus position)
MLTI	mixed lymphocytic-tumor interaction
MLV	Moloney's leukemogenic virus; mouse leukemia virus
MLVP	mean left ventricular pressure
mm.	milli-meter (milli-metre)
mM	milli-mole
M&M	milk and molasses; morbidity and mortality
MM	malignant melanoma; medial malleolus; mucous membrane; multiple myeloma; muscularis mucosa
MMAS	methionine mal-absorption syndrome
MMC	minimal medullary concentration; morbidity and mortality conference
mmCi	milli-micro-Curie
MMD	minimal morbidostatic dose
MMDA	5-methoxy-3,4-methylene-dioxy-amphetamine
MMEF	maximal mid-expiratory flow
MMEF$_{25-75\%}$	mean flow rate during the middle half of the forced expiratory vital capacity
MMEFR	maximal mid-expiratory flow rate
MMEP	multi-modality evoked potential
MMF	mean maximum flow
mmg	milli-micro-gram (nanogram)
mmHg	milli-meters of mercury (milli-metres of mercury)
MMIF	marcophage migration inhibiting factor
MMLV	Moloney murine leukemia virus
MMMT	malignant mixed mesodermal tumor
mmol	milli-mole
mmol/l	milli-mole-liter (milli-mole-litre)
mmol/L	milli-mole-liter (milli-mole-litre)
m.m.p.	mixture melting point

MMPI	Minnesota Multiphasic Personality Inventory
MMPR	methyl-mercapto-purine roboside
MMR	maternal mortality rate; measles, mumps, rubella; midline malignant reticulosis
MMRG	mass miniature radio-graphy
MMRV	measles, mumps, rubella, varicella
MMT	mouse mammary tumor
MMTV	mouse mammary tumor virus
MMV	mandatory minute volume
MMWR	Morbidity and Mortality Weekly Report
mN	milli-normal
Mn	Manganese
M&N	morning and night
MN	Medical News; mid-night; motor neuron; myo-neural
MNC	meatus nasi communis
MNCF	mono-nuclear cell factor
MNCV	motor nerve conduction velocity
mngr.	manager
MNM	meatus nasi medius
MNS	meatus nasi superior
MNU	methyl-nitroso-urea
Mo	Molybdenum; Monday; month; mouth
MO	mail order; main office; main operation; major operation; Medical Officer; mesio-occlusal; mineral oil; money order (bookkeeping abbreviation)
MOB	Methyldiamine, Oncovin, Bleomycin
MOB-P	Mitomycin, Oncovin, Bleomycin, Platinol
MOCA	Methotrexate, Oncovin, Cyclophosphamide, Adriamycin
mod.	*modicus* (moderate); modification; modify
MOD	Manager On Duty; mesio-occluso-distal
MODEM	Modulator-Demodulator
MODM	mature onset diabetes mellitus
MODY	maturity-onset diabetes of youth
MOE	movement of extremities
MOF	MeCCNU, Oncovin, Fluorouracil
mol.	mole; molecule
molal.	molality
mol-c	molar concentration
moll.	*mollis* (soft)
mol. wt	molecular weight
MOM	middle of month; milk of magnesia
MOMP	Mechlorethamine, Oncovin, Methotrexate, Prednisone

Mon.	Monday
monos.	monocytes
MOP	mask of pregnancy; Mechlorethamine, Oncovin, Procarbazine
MOPP	Mechlorethamine, Oncovin, Procarbazine, Prednisone
MOPV	Monovalent Oral Polio virus (Vaccine); Monovalent Oral Polio-virus (Vaccine); Monovalent Oral Poliovirus Vaccine
M.O.R.C.	Medical Officers Reserve Corps
morph.	morphine
mos.	months
mOs	milli-osmol
mOsm	milli-osmol
m.p.	*mane primo* (early in the morning); *massa pilularam* (pill mass); melting point; *modo praescripto* (in the way prescribed)
MP	maculo papules; major part; Melphalan, Prednisone; menstrual period; Mercapto-Purine (Leukerin; Purinethol); mesio-pulpal; metatarso-phalangeal; methyl-prednosolone; mono-phosphate; multi-parous; multi-peace
6-MP	6-Mercapto-Purine (Leukerin; Purinethol)
M.P.A.	Master of Public Administration
MPA	main pulmonary artery; methyl-prednisolone acetate
MPAP	mean pulmonary artery pressure
MPASI	mantle para-aortic splenic irradiation
MPAWP	mean pulmonary artery wedge pressure
MPBS	male pattern baldness scale
MPC	maximum permissible concentration; Meperidine, Promethazine, Chlorpromazine
MPD	maximum permissible dose
MPDE	maximum permissible dose equivalent
MPDS	myofacial pain-dysfunction syndrome
MPFT	moving platform fistula test
MPGA	mean projected gestational age
MPGN	membrano-proliferative glomerulo-nephritis
M.P.H.	Master of Public Health
MPH	meters per hour (metres per hour); miles per hour
MPHR	maximum predicted heart rate
MPI	Myocardial Perfusion Imaging
MPJ	metatarso-phalangeal joint
MPL	maximum permissible level; mesio-pulpo-lingual
MPLa	mesio-pulpo-labial

MPM	meters per minute (metres per minute); miles per minute
MPMV	Mason-Pfizer monkey virus
MPN	most probable number
MPP	mercapto-pyrazido-pyrimidine
mps	meters per second (metres per second); miles per second
MPS	muco-poly-saccharidosis; multi-phasic screening
M-PSEUDO	male pseudohermaphroditism (androgyny; hermaphroditism); *pseudohermaphroditismus masculinus*
MPSS	methyl-prednisolone sodium succinate
MPU	micro-processor unit
MPV	metatarsus primus varus
MPX	multiplex
mR	milli-Roentgen
M&R	measure and record
MR	magnetic resonance; major risk; medial rectus; medical record; medical report; mega-Roentgen; mental retardation; metabolic rate; methyl red; mitral reflux; mitral regurgitation; mortality rate; muscle relaxant
MR×1	may repeat once
MRA	Magnetic Resonance Angiography; Medical Record Administrator
MRAP	mean right atrial pressure
MRC	Medical Research Council; Medical Reserve Corps
MRCP	Member of the Royal College of Physicians
MRCS	Member of the Royal College of Surgeons
MRCVS	Member of the Royal College of Veterinary Surgeons
MRD	minimum reacting dose
MRF	mitral regurgitant flow
MRFIT	Multiple Risk Factor Intervention Trial
MRI	magnetic resonance imaging
MRL	major retaining ligament
MRM	modified radical mastectomy
MRMIB	Major Risk Medical Insurance Board
MRN	malignant renal neoplasm
mRNA	messenger ribo-nucleic acid
MRSA	methicillin-resistant *Staphylococcus aureus*
MRSG	magnetic resonance spectro-graphy
MRSS	magnetic resonance spectro-scopy
MRT	maximum recovery time
MRVP	mean right ventricular pressure
m.s.	milli-second; *more solito* (as accustomed; in the usual way)

ms	milli-second
M.S.	*Scientiae Magister* (Master of Science); Master of Surgery
MS	major surgery; mass spectrometry; Ménière's syndrome; metric scale; metric system; mitral sound; mitral stenosis; morphine sulfate; multiple sclerosis; muscle strength; musculo-skeletal
MS-1	strain of hepatitis virus type 1
MS-2	strain of hepatitis virus type 2
MSA	management service agreement; management services agreement
MSAFP	maternal serum alpha-feto-protein
MSB	most significant bit
MSBOS	maximum surgical blood order schedule
M.Sc.	*Scientiae Magister* (Master of Science)
MSD	menadiol sodium diphosphate; most significant digit
MSDP	menadiol sodium di-phosphate
msec.	milli-second
MSER	mean systolic ejection rate
msg.	massage; message
MSG	mono-sodium glutamate
MSH	melanocyte-stimulating hormone
MSHF	melanocyte-stimulating hormone factor
MSH-IF	melanocyte-stimulating hormone inhibiting factor
MSH-RF	melanocyte-stimulating hormone releasing factor
MSK	mask; medullary sponge kidney
MSL	mid-sternal line; muscle
MSLA	mouse specific lymphocyte antigen
MSLT	multiple sleep latency test
MSO	management services organization
MSOF	multiple system organ failure
MSP	median sagittal plane
MSR	muscle strength reflex; muscle stretch reflex
mss.	manuscripts
MSSA	methicillin-sensitive *Staphylococcus aureus*
MSSU	mid-stream specimen of urine
MST	median survival time; melanocyte-stimulating hormone; Mountain Standard Time
MsTh	meso-thorium
MsTh-1	mesothorium type 1
MsTh-2	mesothorium type 2
MSU	mid-stream urine (specimen); mono-sodium-urate
MSUD	maple syrup urine disease
MSV	Moloney's sarcoma virus; murine sarcoma virus

MSVC	maximal sustained ventilatory capacity
M&T	muscles and tendons
MT	empty; malignant teratoma; Medical Technologist; Medical Transcriptionist; meta-tarsal; mountain; music therapy
MTA	meta-tarsus adductus; Microculture Tetrazolium Assay
MTB	*Mycobacterium tuberculosis*
MTBF	mean time between failures
MTBT	malignant tropho-blastic teratoma
MTC	medullary thyroid carcinoma; minimum toxic concentration
m.t.d.	*mitte tales doses* (send such doses)
MTD	maximally tolerated dose; mean tumor diameter
mtg.	meeting
MTHFA	methyl-tetra-hydro-folic acid
MTI	malignant teratoma intermediate
MTIC	methyl-triazino-imidazole carboxamide
MTJ	mid-tarsal joint
MTP	median time to progression; meta-tarso-phalangeal
MTR	mean total reactivity; meter (metre)
MTS	male Turner's syndrome; Medi-Cal transaction software
MTT	malignant trophoblastic teratoma; mean transit time
MTU	malignant teratoma undifferentiated; methyl-thio-uracil
MTV	mammary tumor virus; meta-tarsus varus
MTX	Methotrexate (Amethopterin)
MTX-BCD	Methotrexate, Bleomycin, Cytoxan, Dactinomycin
MTX-CHOP	Methotrexate, Cytoxan, Hydroxydaunomycin, Oncovin, Prednisone
MTX-LVR	Methotrexate, Leucovorin
MTZ	mono-tetra-zolium
m.u.	mouse unit
mU	milli-unit
MUC	maximum urinary concentration
mucil.	*mucilago* (mucilage)
MuGA	multiple-gated acquisition (scan of heart)
MUGA	multiple-gated acquisition (scan of heart)
multip.	multipara; multiparous; multiple; multiplication; multiply
MUO	metastasis of unknown origin
musc.	muscle; muscles; muscular; masculine
Must.	Mustargen (Mechlorethamine)
MUU	mouse uterine unit
MUX	multiplex; multiplexer; multiplex transmission

mV	milli-volt
Mv	Mendelevium
M.V.	*Medicus Veterinarius* (Veterinary Physician)
MV	mechanical ventilation; mega-volt; mitral valve
MVA	mitral valve area
MVAC	Methotrexate, Vincristine, Adriamycin, Cisplatin
MVC	maximum vital capacity; motor vehicle accident
MVHP	micro-vascular hydrostatic pressure
MVI	multi-vitamin infusion
MVO_2	myocardial ventilation of oxygen (consumption); myocardial ventilation of oxygen (rate)
MVP	Mitomycin C, Velban, Platinol; mitral valve prolapse
MVPP	Mechlorethamine, Velban, Procarbazine, Prednisone
MVR	massive vitreous retraction; maximum ventilation rate; minute volume of respiration; mitral valve replacement
MVV	maximum ventilation volume; maximum voluntary ventilation; measles virus vaccine; Mechlorethamine, Vincristine, Velban
mW	milli-watt
M.W.	molecular weight
MW	mega-watt; mirror writing
MWD	micro-wave diathermy
MWT	Mallory-Weiss tear
MX	mix; mixture; presence of metastasis cannot be assessed
mxd	mixed
my.	myopia
My.	May
myc.	mycology
mycol.	mycology
myop.	myopia
MYXO	myxoma; Myxomycetes; myxorrhea; myxovirus
MZ	mono-zygotic

~ N ~

Ⓝ	notified
n.	nano-; *nervus* (nerve); neutron; *noris* (nostril); normal
N	nasal; nation; national; nausea; needle; negative; Neisseria; nerve; neutron; new; Newton; night; nitrogen; no; node; noise; none; noon; normal; north; nose; note; number; neutron
N_A	Avogadro's number
N_D	refractive index
Na	*Natrium* (sodium)
Na^+	Natrium ion (sodium ion)
N.A.	Nomina Anatomica; numerical aperture
N/A	not applicable
NA	Narcotics Anonymous; neutralizing antibody; not admitted; not applicable; not available; numerical aperture
Na_e	total exchangeable natrium (total exchangeable sodium)
NAA	no apparent abnormalities
NAACLS	National Accrediting Agency for Clinical Laboratory Science
NAACP	National Association for the Advancement of Colored People
$Na_2B_4O_7$	natrium-borate (borax; sodium-borate)
NaBr	natrium-bromide (sodium-bromide)
NABS	National AIDS Behavioral Surveys
NABx	needle aspiration biopsy
NACA	National Advisory Council on Aging
$NaC_2H_3O_2$	natrium-acetate (sodium-acetate)
NACHRI	National Association of Children's Hospitals and Related Institutions
NaCl	natrium-chloride (sodium-chloride = halite)
NaClO	natrium-hypochlorite (sodium-hypochlorite)
$NaClO_3$	natrium-chlorate (sodium-chlorate)
Na_2CO_3	natrium-carbonate (sodium-carbonate; washing soda)
$Na_2C_2O_3$	natrium-oxalate (sodium-oxalate)

NAD	nicotinamide-adenine dinucleotide; no abnormality detected; no active disease; no acute distress; no apparent distress; no appreciable disease
NADL	National Association of Dental Laboratories
NADP	nicotinamide-adenine dinucleotide phosphate
NAEMT	National Association of Emergency Medical Technicians
NaF	natrium-fluoride (sodium-fluoride)
NaHCO$_3$	natrium-bicarbonate (baking soda; sodium-bicarbonate)
NaH$_2$PO$_4$	mononatrium acid phosphate (monosodium acid phosphate)
Na$_2$HPO$_4$	dinatrium acid phosphate (disodium acid phosphate)
NaI	natrium-iodide (sodium-iodide)
NAI	non-accidental injury
NAME	Nevi, Atrial myxoma, Myxoid neurofibroma, Ephilides
NAMH	National Association of Mental Health
NANB-H	non-A, non-B hepatitis
NANB-V	non-A, non-B virus
NANDA	North American Nursing Diagnosis Association
NaNO$_2$	natrium-nitrite (sodium-nitrite)
NANSAID	Non-Aspirin, Non-Steroidal, Anti-Inflammatory Drug
NaOH	natrium-hydroxide (caustic soda; lye soda; sodium-hydroxide)
NAON	National Association of Orthopaedic Nurses
NAOT	National Association of Orthopaedic Technicians
NAPA	N-acetyl-procain-amide
NAPH	National Association of Public Hospitals
NAPNAP	National Association of Pediatric Nurse Associates and Practitioners
NAS	nasal; National Academy of Sciences; no added salt
Na$_2$SO$_4$	natrium-sulfate (Glauber's salt; sodium-sulfate)
Na$_2$S$_2$O$_3$	natrium-thiosulfate (sodium-thiosulfate)
NASW	National Association of Social Workers
NAT	national; natural; no action taken
NAUC	normalized area under curve
n.b.	*nota bene* (note well)
Nb	Niobium
NB	new-born; *nota bene* (note well)
NBI	no body injury; no bone injury
NBL	non-Burkitt's lymphoma
NBM	normal bowel movement; nothing by mouth
NBS	National Bureau of Standards; normal blood serum; normal bowel sounds; normal breath sounds

NBT	nitro-blue tetrazolium (test)
NBTE	non-bacterial thrombotic endocarditis
NBTEc	non-bacterial thrombotic endocarditis
NBW	normal birth weight
N:C	nuclear : cytoplasmic (ratio)
N/C	no charge; nuclear : cytoplasmic (ratio); numerical control
NC	no change; no charge; no complaints; no cost; not cultured
NCA	neuro-circulatory asthenia
NCADI	National Clearinghouse for Alcohol and Drug Information
NCALL	null cell acute lymphocytic leukemia
NCC	natural cytotoxic cell
NCCLS	National Committee for Clinical Laboratory Standards
NCDB	National Cancer Data Base
NCE	non-cardiogenic edema
NCEP	National Cholesterol Education Program
NCF	neutrophil chemotactic factor
NCF-A	neutrophil chemotactic factor of anaphylaxis
NCHLS	National Council of Health Laboratory Services
NCHS	National Center Health Statistics
nCi	nano-Curie
NCI	National Cancer Institute; nuclear contour index
NCI-SPORE	National Cancer Institute's Specialized Programs of Research Excellence
NCMH	National Committee on Mental Hygiene
NCN	National Council of Nurses
NCPCC	National Clearinghouse of Poison Control Centers
NCR	National Case Registry
NCRE	National Council on Rehabilitation Education
NCRP	National Committee on Radiation Protection and Measurements
NCT	neural crest tumor
NCTC	natural cytotoxic T-cell
NCV	nerve conduction velocity; non-cholerea vibrosis
Nd	Neodymium
ND	natural death; Newcastle Disease; no date; no disease; none detected; normal delivery; not detected; not done
NDA	National Dental Association; new drug application; no data available; no demonstrable antibodies
NDDG	National Diabetes Data Group
NDGA	nordi-hydro-guaiaretic acid
NDI	nephrogenic diabetes insipidus

NDIRA	non-dispersive infra-red analysis
NDMA	nitroso-di-methyl-aniline
NDP	net dietary protein
NDR	National Dialysis Registry; no drug reaction
NDV	Newcastle Disease Virus
Ne	Neon
NE	neurologic examination; no effect; non-elastic; not enlarged; not examined
neb.	*nebula* (a spray)
nec.	necessary
NEC	necrotizing entero-colitis; not elsewhere classifiable; not elsewhere classified
NED	no evidence detected; no evidence of disease
NEEP	negative end-expiratory pressure
NEFA	non-esterified fatty acid
neg.	negative
NeGram	nalidixic acid (Dixiben; Uralgin; Urodixin)
NEHA	National Environmental Health Education
NEI	National Eye Institute
NENSG	non-erosive non-specific gastritis
NEO	necrotizing external otitis
NER	nerve; no evidence of recurrence
NERD	no evidence of recurrent disease
nerv.	*nervosus* (nervous); *nervus* (nerve)
NES	not elsewhere specified
NET	naso-endotrachial tube
neuro.	neurological
nF	nano-Farad
NF	National Formulary; non-fiction; not felt; not fixed; not found
NFID	National Foundation for Infectious Diseases
NFLPN	National Federation for Licensed Practical Nurses
NFP	natural family planning
NFTD	normal full-term delivery
ng	nano-gram (milli-micro-gram)
NG	naso-gastric; *Neisseria gonorrhea*; *Neisseria gonorrhoeae*; nitro-glycerin; no gas; not given; no good
NGF	nerve growth factor
NGT	naso-gastric tube
NG tube	naso-gastric tube
NGU	non-gonococcal urethritis
NH	need help; normal heat; nursing home
NH_3	ammonia (am u̅n, Egyptian deity)

NHANES	National Health and Nutrition Examination Surveys
NH_4Br	ammonium-bromide
NHC	National Health Council; non-histiocytic lymphoma
NH_4Cl	ammonium-chloride
NH_4CNO	ammonium-cyanate
$(NH_2)_2CO$	urea (carbamide)
$(NH_4)_2CO_3$	ammonium-carbonate
NHCP	non-histone chromosomal protein
NHF	Nursing History Form
NH_4HS	ammonium-hydrosulfide
NHL	nodular histiocytic lymphoma; non-Hodgkin's lymphoma
NHLBI	National Heart, Lung and Blood Institute
NHLI	National Heart and Lung Institute
NHMRC	National Health and Medical Research Council
NH_4NO_3	ammonium-nitrate
NHO	National Hospice Organization
N.H.S.	National Health Service (British)
NHS	normal human serum; normal horse serum
NHSDA	National Household Survey of Drug Abuse
$(NH_4)_2SO_2$	ammonium-sulfate
Ni	Nickel
NI	no information; not informed; not identified; not investigated; not isolated; no isolation
NIA	National Institute on Aging; nephelometric inhibition assay
NIAAA	National Institute on Alcohol Abuse and Alcoholism
NIAID	National Institute of Allergy and Infectious Diseases
NIAMD	National Institute of Arthritis and Metabolic Diseases
NIAMDD	National Institute of Arthritis, Metabolic and Digestive Diseases
NIAMSD	National Institute of Arthritis, Musculoskeletal and Skin Diseases
NICHHD	National Institute of Child Health and Human Development
NICU	Neonatal Intensive Care Unit
NIDA	National Institute on Drug Abuse
NIDD	non-insulin dependent diabetes
NIDDKD	National Institute for Diabetes, Digestive and Kidney Diseases
NIDDM	non-insulin dependent diabetes mellitus
NIDR	National Institute of Dental Research
NIEHS	National Institute of Environmental Health Sciences

NIERO	non-invasive evaluation of radiation output
nig.	*niger* (black)
NIGMS	National Institute of General Medical Sciences
NIH	National Institutes of Health
NIMH	National Institute of Mental Health
NINCDS	National Institute of Neurological and Communicative Disorders and Stroke
NINDB	National Institute of Neurological Diseases and Blindness
NINDS	National Institute of Neurological Disorders and Stroke
NIOSH	National Institute of Occupational Safety and Health
nitro.	nitrogen; nitroglycerin
NJ	naso-jejunal
NK	natural killer; Nomenklatur Kommission; not known
NKA	no known abnormalities; no known allergies
NKAD	no known allergies to drugs
NKD	no known diseases
NKDA	no known drug allergies
NKH	non-ketotic hyperosmotic
n.l.	*non licet* (it is not lawful); *non liquet* (it is not clear)
nl.	nano-liter (nano-litre)
nL	nano-liter (nano-litre)
NL	norma lateralis; normal; normal link; nasal line
NLA	neuro-lept-analgesia
NLM	National Library of Medicine
NLN	National League for Nursing
NLTT	normal lymphocyte transfer test
n.m.	*nocte maneque* (at night and morning)
nm	nano-meter (nano-metre)
N-m	Newton-meter (Newton-metre)
NM	neuro-muscular; no meat; not measured; nuclear medicine
NMA	National Medical Association; neurogenic muscular atrophy
NMAC	National Minority Aids Council
NMG	N-methyl-gucamine
NMJ	neuro-muscular junction
NMLRC	National Medical Liability Reform Coalition
NMN	nicotinamide mono-nucleotide
nmol.	nano-mole
NMP	normal menstrual period
NMR	nuclear magnetic resonance

NMRI	Naval Medical Research Institute; nuclear magnetic resonance imaging
NMS	neuroleptic malignant syndrome
nn.	*nervi* (nerves)
NNAT	neo-natal alloimmune thrombocytopenia
NNATP	neo-natal alloimmune thrombocytopenia purpura
NND	neo-natal death
NNS	National Natality Survey
NNVD	no neck vein distention
no.	*numero* (number)
No	Nobelium
NO	needs oxygen; nitric oxide; no operation; no output; no oxygen; not obtained; not occupied; not operated
N₂O	nitrous-oxide (dinitrogen-monoxide)
noc.	*nocte* (night)
noc. man.	*nocte maneque* (at night and morning)
non. rep.	*non repetatur* (let it not be repeated)
NOPHN	National Organization for Public Health Nursing
n.o.s.	not otherwise specified
nos.	*numeros* (numbers)
NOS	not otherwise specified
NOSIE	Nurse Observation Scale for Inpatient Evaluation
Nov.	November
nox.	*nocxte* (night)
Np	Neptunium
NP	army medicines; Naptalam; naso-pharyngeal; naso-pharynx; needs priest; nerve palsy; neuro-psychiatric; neuro-psychiatrist; neuro-psychiatry; new patient; nitrogen phosphorus; no pain; no priest; no protest; no pulse; normal plasma; not palpable; not performed; nucleo-protein; Nurse Practitioner; nursing practice
NPA	Naptalam; National Perinatal Association
NPB	nodal premature beat
NPC	naso-pharyngeal carcinoma; National Pharmaceutical Council; nodal premature complex; nodal premature contraction
NPCDP	National Prostatic Cancer Detection Project
NPD	nitrogen phosphorus detector; no pathologic diagnosis
NPDB	National Practitioner Data Bank
NPDL	nodular poorly differentiated lymphocytes
NPDR	non-proliferative diabetic retinopathy
NPDRP	non-proliferative diabetic retino-pathy
NPHC	normal pressure hydro-cephalus

NPH ins.	Neutral Protamine Hagedorn insulin
NPN	non-protein nitrogen
NPNT	non-palpable non-tender
n.p.o.	*nulla per os* (nothing by mouth; nothing per os)
NPO/HS	*nulla per os / hora somni* (nothing by mouth at bedtime)
NPP	nitro-phenyl-phosphate
4-NPP	4-nitro-phenyl-phosphate
NPR	net protein ration
NPSG	nocturnal poly-somno-graphy
NPT	neo-precipitin test; nocturnal penile tumescene; normal pressure and temperature
NPU	net protein utilization
n.r.	*non repetatur* (do not repeat)
NR	negative response; nerve root; nodal rhythm; non-reactive; no radiation; no reaction; no record; no refill; no report; no response; no resuscitation; normal range; normal rhythm; not ready; not recorded; not remarkable; not resolved
NRBC	nucleated red blood cell
NRC	National Research Council; normal retinal correspondence; not responded completely; Nuclear Regulatory Commission
NRCA	National Rehabilitation Counseling Association
NRCC	National Registry in Clinical Chemistry
NRD	non-renal death
NREM	non-rapid eye movement
NREMS	non-rapid eye movement sleep
NREMT	National Registry of Emergency Medical Technicians
NRM	National Registry of Microbiologists
nRNA	nuclear ribo-nucleic acid
NRS	non-reactive system; normal rabbit serum
ns	nano-second
N/S	no standard; normal saline
NS	nasal surgery; need surgery; negative state; nervous system; neuro-surgery; non-specific; normal saline; no salt; no sample; no surgery; no syndrome; not shown; not significant; not specified; not sufficient; nylon suture
NSA	normal serum albumin
NSABP	National Surgical Adjuvant Breast Project
NSAIA	non-steroidal anti-inflammatory analgesic
NSAID	non-steroidal anti-inflammatory drug
NSB	non-specific binding
NSC	no significant change

NSC-8806	Melphalan
NSCFPT	no significant change from previous tracing
NSCLC	non-small cell lung cancer
NSD	nominal single dose; nominal standard dose; non-specifc esterase; normal spontaneous delivery; no significant defect; no significant deviation; no significant difference; no significant disease; no sufficient data
NSE	non-specific enolase
nsec.	nano-second
NSEMD	non-specific esophageal motility disorder
NSF	National Science Foundation
NSFTD	normal spontaneous full-term delivery
NSG	nursing
NSGCT	non-seminomatosus germ cell tumor
NSHCA	non-specific hepato-cellular abnormality
NSHD	nodular sclerosing Hodgkin's disease
NSILA	non-suppressible insulin-like activity
NSNA	National Student Nurse Association
NSND	non-symptomatic non-disabling
NSP1	non-structural protein 1
NSP2	non-structural protein 2
NSR	nasal septal reconstruction; normal sinus rhythm
NSS	normal saline solution
NST	non-shivering thermogenesis; non-stress test; nucleus of solitary tract
NSU	non-specific urethritis
NSV	non-specific vaginitis
NSVD	normal spontaneous vaginal delivery
NSVTC	non-sustained ventricular tachy-cardia
nt.	night
Nt	Niton
N&T	nose and throat
NT	naso-trachial; neural tube; new test; new trainee; no test; not tested
NTA	nitrilo-triacetic acid
NTAB	nephro-toxic anti-body
NTC	nodal tachy-cardia
NTD	neural tube defect
NTE	not to exceed
NTG	nitro-glycerin; non-toxic goiter
NTMI	non-transmural myocardial infarction
NTN	nephro-toxic nephritis
NTP	normal temperature and pressure; nucleoside

	5´-tri-phosphate
NTPP	normal temperature, pressure, and pulse
NTS	not to scale
NTSC	National Television Systems Committee
NTU	nephelometric turbidity units
NTV	nerve tissue vaccine
NTW	network
nt. wt.	net weight
nU	nano-unit
NU	name unknown; new unit; Numorphan; Nupercaine
NUG	necrotizing ulcerative gingivitis
num.	number; numeral; numerous; nummular
nun.	*nunc* (now)
N&V	nausea and vomiting
N/V	nausea and vomiting
NV	negative value; negative variation; nevus vascularis; new value; new virus; norma verticalis
NVA	near visual acuity; no value available
NVD	nausea, vomiting and diarrhea; neck vein distention; new virus detected; Newcastle Virus Disease
NVDS	non-invasive vascular diagnostic studies
NVSD	no vital signs detected
NWDL	nodular well-differentiated lymphocytes
NWG	non-weight bearing
NWGHGT	National Working Group on Human Gene Therapy
nwk.	network
NX	regional lymph nodes cannot be assessed
NYD	not yet diagnosed; not yet done
nyx.	nyxis (paracentesis)
NZ	New Zealand
NZBM	New Zealand black mouse
NZWM	New Zealand white mouse

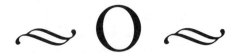

o.	*octarius* (pint); *oculus* (eye)
O	nil; no; none; object; objection; obstruction; occiput; occlusal; occupation; office; oil; Oncovin; open; opened; opening; operation; oral; orally; organ; organic; out; output; oxygen
O_2	oxygen
O_2-ext	oxygen extraction rate
O_3	ozone
o/a	on or about
OA	occipital artery; ocular albinism; osteo-arthritis; oxalic acid
OA-1	ocular albinism type 1
OA-2	ocular albinism type 2
OAA	Opticians Association of America
OAAD	ovarian ascorbic acid depletion
OAD	obstructive airway disease
OAF	osteoclast activating factor
OAL	office administrative law
OAP	Oncovin, Ara-C, Prednisone; osteo-arthro-pathy
OAT	ornithine amino-transferase
OAVD	oculo-auriculo-vertebral dysplasia
OAWO	opening abductory wedge osteotomy
o.b.	*omni bihora* (every 2 hours)
O&B	opium and belladonna
OB	obstetrics; occult blood
Obc.	obcecation
Obd.	obdormition; obduction
OBG	obstetrics and gynecology
OB/GYN	obstetrics and gynecology
obj.	object; objection
OBRA	Omnibus Budget Reconciliation Act
OBS	observation; observe; observed; organic brain syndrome
obst.	obstetric; obstruction
OBT	occult blood test

o.c.	*opus citatum* (in the work cited)
Oc.	occupation; October; octyl
OC	object choice; occluso-cervical; office call; on call; *Onchocerca caecutiens*; operative cholecystectomy; oral contraceptive; organic chemistry
OCA	oculo-cutaneous albinism
occ.	occasional; occipital; occiput
OCCG	oral chole-cysto-gram
OCG	oral cholecysto-gram
OCP	obsessive-compulsive personality; oral contraceptive pill
OCR	optical character recognition
Oct.	October
OCT	ornithine carbamoyl-transferase; oxytocin challenge test
O.D.	Doctor of Optometry; *oculus dexter* (right eye); *omni die* (every day); outside diameter; over-dose
OD	occupational dermatosis; occupational disease; over-dose
ODA	occipito-dextra anterior (fetus position)
ODC	oxygen dissociation curve
OD'd	overdosed
ODDD	oculo-dendo-digital dysplasia
ODM	ophthalmo-dynamo-metry
ODO	oculo-dento-osseous
ODP	occipito-dextra posterior (fetus position)
ODQ	opponens digiti quinti
ODT	occipito-dextra transversa (fetus position)
o.e.	omissions excepted
O&E	observation and examination
OE	olfactory esthesioneuroma; ophthalmoplegia externa; oral examination; otitis externa
OEF	occipital eye field
OER	oxygen enhancement ratio
OES	oral erotic stage
OF	occipital frontal; *Opisthorchis felineus*
OFA	onco-fetal antigen
OFAGE	Orthogonal Field Agarose Gel Electrophoresis
ofc.	office
OFC	occipito-frontal circumference
OFD	object film distance; ora-facio-digital; oral facial digital
OFT	osmotic fragility test
OG	obstetrics and gynecology

OGF	oxygen gain factor
OGTT	oral glucose tolerance test
o.h.	*omni hora* (at every hour)
OH	hydroxyl
17-OHCS	17-hydroxy-cortico-steroid
OHD	organic heart disease
25-OHD$_3$	vitamin D
OHL	oral hairy leucoplakia (leukoplakia)
OHP	oxygen at high pressure
17-OHP	17-hydroxy-progesterone
OHT	ocular hyper-tension
OI	ophthalmoplegia interna; opportunistic infection; os ilium; osteogenesis imperfecta
OIC	osteogenesis imperfecta congenita
OID	object image distance
OIG	Office of Inspector General
OIH	ortho-iodo-hippurate
OIMD	optimal immuno-modulating dose
OJ	organ of Jacobson
OK	all right; approve; opto-kinetics; authorize
OK-432	Picibanil
OKN	opto-kinetic nystagmus
o.l.	*oculus laevus* (left eye)
ol.	*oleum* (oil)
OLA	occipito-laeva anterior (fetus position)
OLC	obstructive lung chronic
OLD	obstructive lung disease
OLH	ovine lactogenic hormone
ol. oliv.	*oleum olivae* (olive oil)
OLP	occipito-laeva posterior (fetus position)
OLT	occipito-laeva transversa (fetus position)
o.m.	*omni mane* (on every morning)
OM	obtuse marginal (coronary artery); occipito-mental; occupational medicine; onychia maligna; orbito-meatal; osteo-myelitis; otitis media
OMB1	obtuse marginal branch — first
OMB2	obtuse marginal branch — second
om. bid.	*omnibus bidendis* (every 2 days)
om. bih.	*omni bihoris* (every second hour)
OMCI	old myo-cardial infarction
OMD	ocular muscle dystrophy
OMDA	Oncovin, Methotrexate, Doxorubicin, Actinomycin D

OME	otitis media effusion
om. hor.	*omni hora* (every hour)
OMM	ophthalmo-mandibulo-melic
om. noc.	*omni nocte* (every night)
OMPA	octa-methyl-pyrophosphor-amide; otitis media, purulent, acute
OMS	Organic Mental Syndrome
o.m.v.n.	*omni mane vel nocte* (every morning or night)
o.n.	*omni nocte* (every night)
ON	olfactory nerves; optic nerve; Orthopedic Nurse
ONA	Oncology Nurses Association
OND	optic nerve disease
o.o.	*oleum olivae* (olive oil)
OOB	out of bed
OOC	organ of Corti
O&P	ova and parasites
OP	occiput posterior; onychia parasitica; opening pressure; operation; operative procedure; osmotic pressure; out-patient
OPC	out-patient clinic; overall performance category
OPD	out-patient department
OPDS	otopalato-digital syndrome
OPF	omental pedicle flap; operative pedicle flap
OPG	ocular plethysmo-graphy; ocular pressure gradient; oxy-poly-gelatin
ophth.	ophthalmology
OPL	Oncovin, Prednisone, Leucogen
OPM	occult primary malignancy
opp.	opposed; opposite; opposition
OPP	Oncovin, Procarbazine, Prednisone
OPPG	oculo-pneumo-plethysmo-graphy
OPRT	oratate-phospho-ribosyl-transferase
OPS	out-patient surgery
opt.	*optimus* (best; optimum)
OPT	out-patient treatment
OPTACON	Optical Tactile Converter
OPV	oral poliomyelitis virus vaccine; oral poliovirus vaccine
o.q.r.	*omni quadrantae horae* (every quarter of an hour); *omni quadrante hora* (every quarter of an hour)
OR	odd ratio; operating-room; oral; orange; over-reaction
orchi.	orchidopexy; orchidotomy; orchiopexy
ord.	order; ordinal; ordinary

ORD	optical rotatory dispersion
ORF	open reduction fixation
org.	organic; organization; organize
ORIF	open reduction and internal fixation
orig.	original
ORL	oto-rhino-laryngology
Orn.	ornithine
Oro.	orotidine
ORS	Orthopaedic Research Society
ORT	operating room technician
ortho.	orthopaedic (orthopedic)
os	*os* (mouth)
Os	Osmium
O.S.	*oculus sinister* (left eye)
OS	objective sign; office surgery; opening snap; operating system; overall survival
OS/2	Operating System / 2
OSA	obstructive sleep apnea
OSAS	obstructive sleep apnea syndrome
OSE	ovarian surface epithelium
OSHA	Occupational Safety and Health Administration
osm.	osmole
OSMED	oto-spondylo-mega-epiphyseal dysplasia
oss.	osseous
osteo.	osteopathy
OT	Occupational Therapist; occupational therapy; old term; old tuberculin; organoleptic test; original tuberculin; orto-tracheal; os trigonum (triangular bone); over-time; oxygen tent
OTC	over-the-counter
OTD	organ tolerance dose
OTO	otology; otomycosis; otopolypus; otoscope; otoscopy
OTR	Ovarian Tumor Registry
OT/RCF	oxygen transport / red cell flow (ratio)
O.U.	*oculus uterque* (each eye); *oculi unitas* (both eyes)
OURQ	outer upper right quadrant
OV	office visit; ovary
OVD	occlusal vertical dimension
O/W	oil / water (ratio)
OW	open wedge; over-weight
OWB	open wedge biopsy
OWL	out of wed-lock

OWR	Oster-Weber-Rendu
OWS	over-wear syndrome
OxPhos.	oxidative phosphorous
OXPHOS	oxidative phosphorous
Oxy.	oxyopia; oxyphonia; Oxyuris
oz.	ounce (French: unce = a twelfth; Latin: *uncia* = a twelfth)
oze.	ozaena; ozena
ozo.	ozone; ozonide; ozostomia

∼ P ∼

^{32}P	phosphorus 32
$\overline{p}$	*post* (after)
P	page; parent; part; passive; past; pathology; patient; peak; periodic; Persian; pharmacopeia; phosphate; phosphorus; physician; pink; plasma; Plasmodium; Platinol; pleura; poise; Portugal; Portuguese; position; post; power; presbyopia; prescription; pressure; priest; print; probability; protein; Proteus; pulmonary; pulpal; pulse; pupil; purple
P_1	pulmonic first sound
P_2	pulmonic second sound
P_B	barometric pressure
P_L	transpulmonary pressure
P_{NA}	plasma sodium
P_{ss}	plasma steady-state concentration
p.a.	*pars affecta* (the part affected); *partes aequales* (equal parts); *partibus aequalibus* (in equal parts)
Pa	Pascal; Protactinium
P&A	percussion and auscultation
P.A.	Physician's Assistant
PA	paralysis agitans; pernicious anemia; phenyl-alanine; posterior artery; postero-anterior; pre-albumin; pre-amplifier; pregnancy associated; primary amenorrhea; primary anemia; pulmonary artery; pulpo-axial
p.a.a.	*parti affectae applicetur* (let it be applied to the affected part)
PAB	premature atrial beat
PABA	para-amino-benzoic acid
PABP	pulmonary artery balloon pump
PAC	Pacific; pacifier; papular acrodermatitis of childhood; Platinol, Adriamycin, Cytoxan; premature atrial complex; premature atrial contraction; premature auricular contraction
PACE	Physician Access and Communication Exchange

$PaCO_2$	arterial carbon dioxide tension
$PACO_2$	alveolar carbon dioxide tension
PACU	post-anesthesia care unit
PAD	pulsating assist device
PADP	pulmonary artery diastolic pressure
PAE	post-antibiotic effect
PAEDP	pulmonary artery end-diastolic pressure
PAF	paroxysmal atrial fibrillation; paroxysmal atrial flutter; platelet activating factor
PAFD	percutaneous abscess and fluid drainage
PAG	peri-aqueductal gray; pregnancy-associated glycoprotein
PAGE	poly-acrylamide gel electrophoresis
PAGT	potential abnormality of glucose tolerance; previous abnormality of glucose tolerance
PAHA	para-amino-hippuric acid
PAHO	Pan American Health Organization
PAHT	pulmonary artery hyper-tension
P-AIDS	pediatric acquired immuno-deficiency syndrome
P-AJCC	Pathological — American Joint Committee on Cancer
PAL	posterior axillary line
palp.	palpable; palpation
PALS	peri-arterial lymphoid sheath
PAM	Melphalan; phenyl-alanine mustard; pulmonary alveolar microlithiasis; Pulse Amplitude Modulation
2-PAM	Pralidoxime (Protopam)
PAN	peri-arteritis nodosa; periodic alternating nystagmus; peroxy-acetyl-nitrate; poly-arteritis nodosa
PAO	peak acid output
PaO_2	alveolar oxygen tension; arterial oxygen tension
PAOD	peripheral arterial occlusive disease
PAOP	pulmonary artery occlusion pressure
pap.	*pappa* (infant's sound for food)
PAP	Papanicolaou (test); passive aggressive personality; peroxidase-anti-peroxidase; positive airway pressure; primary atypical pneumonia; prostatic acid phosphatase; pulmonary alveolar proteinosis; pulmonary artery pressure
PAPP	pregnancy-associated plasma proteins
PAPP-A	pregnancy-associated plasma protein A
PAPS	phospho-adenosyl-phospho-sulfate
Pap smear	Papanicolaou's smear
PAPVC	partial anomalous pulmonary venous connection
PAPVR	partial anomalous pulmonary venous return

PAR	pulmonary arteriolar resistance
PARA	number of viable births (from Latin: *parere* = to give birth)
PARA 0	nulli-para (not delivered a living child)
PARA 1	uni-para (prima-para = for the first time pregnant)
PARA 2	bi-para (secundi-para = for the second time pregnant)
PARA 3	tri-para (for the third time pregnant)
part. aeq.	*partes aequales* (equal parts)
part. vic.	*partitus vicibus* (individual doses)
parv.	*parvus* (small)
PAS	para-amino-salicylic acid; periodic acid-Schiff (reaction); peripheral access system; peripheral anterior synechia; post-anesthesia shivering; pulmonary artery stenosis
PASA	para-amino-salicylic acid
PASG	pneumatic anti-shock garment
PASR	periodic acid-Schiff reaction
PAT	paroxysmal atrial tachycardia; prism adaptation test
PATC	paroxysmal atrial tachy-cardia
PATCO	Prednisone, Ara-C, Thioguanine, Cytoxan, Oncovin
Path.	pathergasia; pathogenic; pathologic; pathology; pathosis
PAV	percutaneous aortic valvuloplasty
PA view	postero-anterior view (X-ray position)
PAW	pulmonary artery wedge
PAWP	pulmonary artery wedge pressure
Pb	*Plumbum* (lead)
PB	paraffin bath; peroneus brevis; pheno-barbital; play-back; protein-bound; pulpo-buccal
PBA	prolactin-binding assay; pulpo-bucco-axial
PBC	primary biliary cirrhosis
P&B exam	pap and breast examination
PBF	pulmonary blood flow
PBG	pedo-baro-graph; porpho-bilino-gen
PBI	protein-bound iodine
PBL	peripheral blood lymphocyte
PBMC	peripheral blood mononuclear cells
PBMM	pedo-baro-macro-meter
PBMNC	peripheral blood mono-nuclear cells
PBN	paralytic brachial neuritis
$Pb(NO_3)_2$	plumbum-nitrate (lead-nitrate)
pbo.	*placebo* (I shall please)
PbO	plumbum-monooxide (lead-monoxide)
PBO	penicillin in beeswax ointment

PBP	penicillin-binding protein
PBPI	penile brachial pressure index
PbS	plumbum-sulfide (lead-sulfide)
PBS	phosphate buffered saline
$PbSO_4$	plumbum-sulfate (lead-sulfate)
PbTe	plumbum-telluride (lead-telluride)
PBT_4	protein-bound thyroxine
PBV	Platinol, Bleomycin, Velban; predicted blood volume; pulmonary blood volume
PBVI	pulmonary blood volume index
PBVP	percutaneous balloon valvulo-plasty
PBW	posterior bite wing
PBX	punch biopsy
PBZ	phenyl-buta-zone
p.c.	*post cibum* (after meals)
pC	pico-Curie
P.C.	Pondus Civile (avoirdupois weight)
PC	packed cells; palmitoyl carnitine; palpebral cartilages; paracentesis cordis; parachordal cartilage; *partus caesareus* (delivery by cesarean section); penis captivus; pentose cycle; personal computer; phosphate cycle; phosphatidyl choline; phospho-creatine; platelet concentrate; Platinol, Cytoxan; present complaint; printed circuit; professional component; professional computer; pulmonary capillary; pulmonic closure; pulse-count
PCA	passive cutaneous anaphylaxis; patient-controlled analgesia; posterior cerebral artery; posterior communicating artery
PCAD	premature coronary artery disease
PCAG	percutaneous carotid arterio-graphy
PCAT	Pharmacy College Admission Test
PCB	para-cervical block
PCBP	poly-chlorinated bi-phenyl
PCC	poison control center; primary care center
PCCM	primary care case managed
PCD	phosphate-citrate-dextrose; poly-cystic disease; posterior corneal deposits; pulmonary clearance delay
PCE	patient care evaluation; pulmo-cutaneous exchange; pyrometric cone equivalent
PCF	posterior cranial fossa
PCG	phono-cardio-gram
PCHU	paroxysmal cold hemoglobin-urea

pCi	pico-Curie
PCI	prophylactic cranial irradiation
PCM	Pulse-Code Modulation
PCMN	protein calorie mal-nutrition
PCN	penicillin
PCNA	proliferating cell nuclear antigen
PCNB	quintozene
PCO	poly-cystic ovary
pCO_2	partial pressure of carbon dioxide; partial tension of carbon dioxide
PCOS	poly-cystic ovarian syndrome
PCP	penta-chloro-phenol; phenyl-cyclohexyl-piperidine; *Pneumocystis carinii* pneumonia; pulmonary capillary pressure
PCPA	para-chloro-phenyl-alanine
PCPBS	Fenson
PCR	polymerase chain reaction
PCS	pieces; porta-caval shunt
pct.	percentage
PCT	porphyria cutanea tarda; porta-caval transposition; prothrombin consumption time
PCTH	porphyria cutanea tarda hereditaria
PCTS	porphyria cutanea tarda symptomatica
PCU	Primary Care Unit
PCV	packed cell volume; poly-chlorinated vinyl; poly-cythemia vera; Procarbazine, Cytoxan, Velban
PCVP	Procarbazine, Cytoxan, Vinblastine, Prednisone
PCW	pulmonary capillary wedge
PCWP	pulmonary capillary wedge pressure
PCx	periscopic convex
PCZ	Procarbazine
Pd	Palladium
P.D.	Doctor of Pharmacy (Pharmacy Doctor)
PD	Parkinson's disease; Pediatric Department; Pediatric Doctor; pediatric dosage; peritoneal dialysis; permanent disability; plasma defect; Police Department; postural drainage; potential difference; Private Detective; professional discount; pulpo-distal; pupillary distance
PDA	pancreatic-duct-arcade; Parenteral Drug Association; patent ductus arteriosus; posterior descending artery; predicted drift angle
PDAB	para-dimethyl-amino-benzaldehyde
PDAC	poorly differentiated adeno-carcinoma

PDC	poorly differentiated carcinoma
PDD	percentage depth dose; pyridoxine deficient diet
PDE	paroxysmal dyspnea on exertion; phospho-di-esterase
PDGF	platelet-derived growth factor
PDI	periodontal disease index
PDL	poorly differentiated lymphocytes
PDLL	poorly differentiated lymphocytic lymphoma
PDMN	poorly differentiated malignant neoplasm
PDP	postural drainage and percussion
PDQ	Physician Data Query
PDR	Physicians' Desk Reference
PDT	photo-dynamic therapy
PE	pelvic examination; paper electrophoresis; potential energy; physical examination; piecemeal excision (of tumor); Platinol, Etoposide; pleural effusion; pharyngo-esophageal; phosphate excretion; physical education; poly-ethylene; pulmonary edema; pulmonary embolism
PEA	phosphotidyl-ethanol-amine; pulseless electrical activity
PEAP	positive end-airway pressure
peds.	pediatrics
PEEP	positive end-expiratory pressure
PEF	peak expiratory flow
PEFR	peak expiratory flow rate
PEG	percutaneous endoscopic gastrostomy; pneumo-encephalography; poly-ethylene glycol
PEGT	percutaneous endoscopic gastrostomy tube
PEL	permissible exposure limit
PEMA	phenyl-ethyl-malon-amide
PEMF	pulsating electro-magnetic field
PEMM	polio-encephalo-meningo-myelitis
pen.	penicillin
PEN	pharmacy equivalent name
PENMT	phospho-ethanolamine-N-methyl transferase
PENS	percutaneous electrical nerve stimulation
PEO	progressive external ophthalmoplegia
PEP	phospho-enol-pyruvate; pre-ejection period; pre-ejection phase
PEPP	positive expiratory pressure plateau
per	*per* (by; per; through)
PER	pronation external rotation; protein efficiency ratio
perf.	perfication; perforated; perforation; performed; perfusion
PERLA	Pupils Equal, Reactive to Light and Accommodation

per os	*per os* (by mouth)
PERRLA	Pupils Equal, Round, Reactive to Light and Accommodation
PERT	Program Evaluation and Review Technique
per vag.	*per vaginam* (through the vagina)
PES	pre-excitation syndrome
PET	petroleum; piecemeal excision of tumor; poly-ethylene terephthalate; positron emission tomography
PETCO$_2$	pressure of end-tidal carbon-dioxide
PETN	penta-erythrityl-tetra-nitrate
PETG	positron emission tomography
PETT	positron emission transaxial tomography
PETTG	positron emission transaxial tomo-graphy
PE tube	ventilating tube for eardrum
pF	pico-Farad
PF	peritoneal fluid; phase factor; plain film; platelet factor; positive factor; posterior fusion; protection factor
PFC	persistent fetal circulation; plaque forming cell
PFD	persistent fetal dispersion
PFFD	proximal focal femoral deficiency
PFIB	per-fluoro-iso-butylene
PFK	phospho-fructo-kinase
PFNAP	percutaneous fine-needle aspiration biopsy
PFP	platelet free plasma
PFR	peak flow rate
PFS	primary fibromyalgia syndrome
PFT	para-fascicular thalamotomy; posterior fossa tumor; pulmonary function test
PFU	plaque forming unit
pg	page; pico-gram
PG	para-genital; para-glossia; pepsino-gen; Pharmacopoeia Germanica; phosphatidyl-glycerol; pituitary gonadotropin; prosta-glandin
PG-I	pepsinogen I
PG-II	pepsinogen II
PGA	prosta-glandin A; pteroyl-glutamic acid (folic acid)
PGA$_1$	prosta-glandin A$_1$
PGA$_2$	prosta-glandin A$_2$
PGA$_3$	prosta-glandin A$_3$
PGB	prosta-glandin B
PGB$_1$	prosta-glandin B$_1$
PGB$_2$	prosta-glandin B$_2$
PGC	prosta-glandin C

PGC_1	prosta-glandin C_1
PGC_2	prosta-glandin C_2
PGC_3	prosta-glandin C_3
PGD	phospho-gluconate dehydrogenase; prosta-glandin D
PGD_1	prosta-glandin D_1
PGD_2	prosta-glandin D_2
PGDR	plasma-glucose disappearance rate
PGE	prosta-glandin E
PGE_1	prosta-glandin E_1
PGE_2	prosta-glandin E_2
PGF	prosta-glandin F
PGF_1	prosta-glandin F_1
PGF_2	prosta-glandin F_2
PGF_{1a}	prosta-glandin F_{1alpha}
PGF_{2a}	prosta-glandin F_{2alpha}
PGF_3	prosta-glandin F_3
PGF_M	prosta-glandin $F_{metabolite}$
PGG_2	prosta-glandin G_2
PGH	pituitary growth hormone; prosta-glandin H
PGH_2	prosta-glandin H_2
PGI	prosta-glandin I; phospho-gluco-isomerase; potassium, glucose, insulin
PGI_2	prosta-glandin I_2
PGK	phospho-glycerate kinase
PGLP	persistent generalized lymphadenopathy
pgm	pico-gram
PGM	phospho-gluco-mutase
PGOS	ponto-geniculo-occiput spike
PGR	psycho-glavanic response
pgs.	pages
PGU	post-gonococcal urethritis
ph.	phalanx; pharmacopoeia (pharmacopeia); phenyl; physics
pH	potential of hydrogen (hydrogen-ion concentration)
PH	patient healh; past history; prostatic hypertrophy; public health
Ph^1	Philadelphia chromosome
PHA	phyto-hem-agglutinin; pulse height analyzer
PHAA	phyto-hem-agglutinin antigen
phar.	pharmaceutical; pharmacist; pharmacy
Phar.B.	*Pharmaciae Baccalaureus* (Bachelor of Pharmacy)
Phar.C.	Pharmaceutical Chemist

Phar.D.	*Pharmaciae Doctor* (Doctor of Pharmacy)
Phar.M.	*Pharmaciae Magister* (Master of Pharmacy)
Ph.B.	*Philosophiae Baccalaureus* (Bachelor of Philosophy); British Pharmacopoeia (Pharmacopeia)
PHBB	propyl-hydroxy-benzyl benzimidazole
Ph.C.	Pharmaceutical Chemist
PHCPP	per-hydro-cyclo-pentano-phenanthrene
Ph.D.	*Philosophiae Doctor* (Doctor of Philosophy)
phenyl.	phenylalanine
Ph ex	physical examination
Ph.G.	Graduate in Pharmacy; Pharmacopoeia Germanica
Ph.I.	International Pharmacopoeia (Pharmacopeia)
PHI	phospho-hexo-isomerase
phial.	*phiala* (bottle)
PHK	phospho-hexo-kinase
PHLLA	post-heparin lipo-lytic activity
PHLPL	post-heparin lipo-protein lipase
PHM	posterior hyaloid membrane
PHN	post-herpetic neuralgia
PHO	Physician-Hospital Organization
pH$_2$O	partial pressure of water vapor
PHP	prepaid health plan
PHPC	pneumo-hemo-peri-cardium
PHPPV	persistent hyper-plastic primary vitreous
PHS	Public Health Service
PHT	pulmonary hypertension
phx.	pharynx
PHx	past history
phys.	physical; physician; physics; physiological
PI	para-influenza; peak index; periodontal index; pili incarnati; present illness; protamine insulin; pulmonary incompetence; pulmonary infarction; pulmonary insufficiency
PIA	plasma insulin activity
PIABCP	percutaneous intra-aortic balloon counter-pulsation
PIC	peripherally inserted catheter; picrol; picture; polymorphism information content
PICA	posterior inferior cerebellar artery; posterior inferior communicating artery
PICU	Pediatric Intensive Care Unit; Pulmonary Intensive Care Unit
PID	pelvic-inflammatory disease; poison ivy dermatitis

PIDT	plasma iron disappearance time
PIE	pulmonary infiltrate with eosinophilia; pulmonary interstitial edema; pulmonary interstitial emphysema
PIF	peak inspiratory flow; prolactin inhibiting factor; proliferation inhibiting factor
PIFR	peak inspiratory flow rate
PIH	pregnancy-induced hypertension
PIHT	pregnancy-induced hyper-tension
pil.	*pilula* (pill); *pilulae* (pills)
PIM	Postgraduate Institute of Medicine
PIN	penile intraepithelial neoplasia; prostatic intraepithelial neoplasia
PINS	persons in need of supervision
PIOPED	prospective investigation of pulmonary embolism diagnosis
PIP	peak inspiratory pressure; proximal inter-phalangeal
PIPJ	proximal inter-phalangeal joint
PIT	patellar inhibition test; plasma iron transfer; plasma iron turnover; prothrombin inhibition test
PITC	phenyl-iso-thio-cyanat
PITR	plasma iron transfer rate; plasma iron turnover rate
PIV	para-influenza virus
PJC	Price-Jones curve; premature junctional contraction
pk.	peak
PK	pain-killer; psycho-kinesis; pyruvate kinase
PKD	polycystic kidney disease
PKP	penetrating kerato-plasty
PKS	pyruvic kinase screening
PKT	packet; pocket; psycho-kinesis test
PKU	phenyl-keton-uria
pKV	peak kilo-voltage
PKV	killed poliomyelitis vaccine
pl.	place; plate; platelet; plural
PL	partial light; partial loss; penis lunatus; perception of light; phantom limb; place; placebo; placental; placental lactogen; pulpo-lingual
PLA	pulpo-linguo-axial
PLAP	peripheral laser angio-plasty; placental alkaline phosphatase
plats.	platelets
PLD	potentially lethal damage
PLDR	potentially lethal damage repair
PLED	periodic lateralized epileptiform discharge

PLEVA	Pityriasis Lichenoides Et Varioliformis Acute
PLF	peri-lymphatic fistula
PLIF	posterior lumbar interbody fusion
PLL	pro-lymphocytic leukemia
PLM	periodic limb movement
PLMs	periodic limb movements
PLSS	portable life support system
PLT	platelet; primed lymphocyte test; primed lymphocyte typing; psittacosis lymphogranuloma venereumtrachoma
PLTS	platelets
PLUVA	psoraline and long-wave ultra-violet A
PLV	live poliomyelitis vaccine; pan-leukopenia virus; phenylalanine lysine vasopressin; posterior left ventricle
p.m.	petit mal; *post meridiem* (afternoon); *post mortem* (autopsy; following death; post-mortem)
pm	pico-meter (pico-metre)
Pm	Promethium
PM	pace-maker; petit mal; Phase Modulation; polymyositis; post-mortem; pulpo-mesial
PMA	para-methoxy-amphetamine; Pharmaceutical Manufacturers Association; progressive muscular atrophy
PMB	post-menopausal bleeding
PMBL	poly-morphonuclear basophil leukocyte
PMBV	percutaneous mitral balloon valvotomy
PMBVP	percutaneous mitral balloon valvulo-plasty
PMC	pre-menstrual change; pseudo-membranous colitis
PMD	personal medical doctor; primary muscular dystrophy; primary myocardial disease; progressive muscular dystrophy
PMDD	pre-menstrual dysphoric disorder
PMEL	poly-morphonuclear eosinophil leukocyte
PMF	Platinol, Mitomycin C, Fluorouracil; progressive massive fibrosis
PMFLEP	progressive multi-focal leuko-encephalo-pathy
PMHx	past medical history
PMI	patient medical instruction; point of maximal impulse; point of maximal intensity; posterior myocardial infarction
PMJC	pre-mature junctional contraction
PML	poly-morphous light; progressive multifocal leukoencephalopathy
PMLE	poly-morphous light eruption
PMM	penta-methyl-melamine

PMMA	poly-methyl-methacrylate augmentation
PMN	poly-morpho-nuclear
PMNBL	poly-morpho-nuclear basophil leukocyte
PMNEL	poly-morpho-nuclear eosinophil leukocyte
PMNL	poly-morpho-nuclear leukocyte
PMNN	poly-morpho-nuclear neutrophil
PMNNL	poly-morpho-nuclear neutrophil leukocyte
PMP	previous menstrual period
PMQ	pyri-methamine-quinine
PM&R	Physical Medicine and Rehabilitation
PMR	perinatal morbidity rate; perinatal mortality rate; poly-morphic reticulosis; proportionate morbidity rate; proportionate mortality rate
PMS	post-menopausal syndrome; post-menstrual stress; pregnant mare's serum; pre-menstrual syndrome
PMSG	pregnant mare serum gonadotropin
PMT	pre-menstrual tension
PMV	prolapse mitral valve
P&N	psychiatry and neurology
PN	percussion note; periarteritis nodosa; peripheral nerve; pneumonia; poly-neuritis; positive-negative; post-natal; progress note
pN_2	partial pressure of nitrogen
PNC	penicillin; premature nodal complex; premature nodal contraction
PND	paroxysmal nocturnal dyspnea; post-nasal drainage; post-nasal drip; pound
PNET	peripheral neuro-ectodermal tumor
PNHU	paroxysmal nocturnal hemoglobin-uria
PNI	psycho-neuro-immunology
PNMT	phosphoethanolamine-N-methyl transferase
PNP	para-nitro-phenol; Pediatric Nurse Practitioner; peripheral neuropathy; psychogenic nocturnal polydipsia
PNPB	positive-negative pressure breathing
PNPP	para-nitro-phenyl-phosphate
PNPS	partial non-progressing stroke
PNS	peripheral nervous system
PNU	protein nitrogen unit
PNVX	pneumococcus vaccine
PNX	pneumothorax
p.o.	*per os* (by mouth)
p/o	post-operative

Po	Polonium
PO	post-operative; pulse-output
pO_2	partial pressure of oxygen; partial tension of oxygen
POA	pancreatic oncofetal antigen; prolapse of anus
POAG	primary open-angle glaucoma
POAH	pre-optical anterior of hypothalamus
POB	phen-oxy-benzamine; place of birth
POC	post-operative care
POCC	Procarbazine, Oncovin, Cytoxan, CCNU
pocil.	*pocillum* (small cup)
pocul.	*poculum* (cup)
POD	post-operative day; pyloric obstruction and dilatation
POEMS	Polyneuropathy, Organomegaly, Endocrinopathy, Monoclonal gammopathy, Skin change
POFA	pancreatic onco-fetal antigen
POG	Pediatric Oncology Group
pOH	potential of hydroxide ion (hydroxide ion concentration)
POHS	presumed ocular histoplasmosis syndrome
POI	prolapse of iris
pol.	poliosis; pollen; pollenosis; pollicization; pollution
POL	Physician Office Laboratory; Poland; Polish
polio.	poliomyelitis; poliosis
poly.	polymorphonuclear leukocyte
POM	Prayer of Maimonides
POMC	pro-opio-melano cortin
POMP	Purinethol, Oncovin, Methotrexate, Prednisone
POMR	problem-oriented medical record
pond.	*pondere* (by weight); *ponderosus* (heavy)
P.OP	post-operative
POP	plasma oncotic pressure; plaster of Paris; post-operative
POPRAS	Problem-Oriented Perinatal Risk Assessment System
POR	pelvic outlet reconstruction; Portugal; Portuguese; problem-oriented record; prolapse of rectum
PORP	partial ossicular reconstructive prosthesis; partial ossicular replacement prosthesis
PORT	portogram; portography; Portugal; Portuguese
PORTO	portogram; portography; portovenogram
POS	periosteal osteo-sarcoma; point of service; position; positive
POSCH	program on the surgical control of hyperlipidemias
post cib.	*post cibum* (after meals)
postop.	post-operation; post-operative

POU	placenta, ovary, uterus; prolapse of uterus
p.p.	*post partum* (after birth); *post prandium* (after meals); *punctum proximum* (near point of accommodation)
pp	pages
P-P	prothrombin — proconvertin
PP	pancreatic polypeptide; partial pressure; pellagra preventive; pelvic peritonectomy; peripheral pulse; pink puffers; posterior pituitary; post-partum; post-prandial; post-puberal; proto-porphia; proximal phalanx; pulse pressure
p.p.a.	*phiala prius agitata* (the bottle being first shaken)
PP&A	palpation, percussion, and auscultation
PPA	phenyl-propanol-amine; phenyl-pyruvic acid
PPAC	Participating Physicians Advisory Council
PPAHN	persistent pulmonary artery hypertension of newborn
PPB	platelet poor blood; positive pressure breathing
PPBS	post-prandial blood sugar
PPC	post-operative pulmonary complication; progressive patient care; protamine para-coagulation
pp'd	postponed; prepared
PPD	packs per day; para-phenylene-diamine; postponed; purified protein derivative (used in Mantoux test)
PPD-S	purified protein derivative — standard
PPF	pellagra preventive factor; plasma protein fraction
ppg	pico-pico-gram
PPH	post-partum hemorrhage; primary pulmonary hypertension
PPHK	platelet phospho-hexo-kinase
PPHPT	pseudo-pseudo-hypo-para-thyroidism
PPHT	primary pulmonary hyper-tension
PPLO	pleuro-pneumonia-like organism
p.p.m	parts per million
PPM	permanent pace-maker; physician-performed microscopy
PPMMA	post-polio-myelitis muscular atrophy
PPN	peripheral parenteral nutrition
PPNG	penicillin-producing *Neisseria gonorrhoeae*
PPO	Preferred Provider Organization; principles and practices of oncology
$P_{50}PO_2$	oxygen tension for producing 50% saturation of hemoglobin
PPP	pancreatic poly-peptide; percusor poly-protein; platelet-poor plasma

PPPPPP	Pain, Pallor, Paresthesia, Pulselessness, Paralysis, Prostration
PPQ bar	pterygo-palato-quadrate bar
PPRC	Physician Payment Review Commission
PPRF	paramedian pontine reticular formation
PPS	pasteurized protein solution; pentosan poly-sulfate; peripheral pulmonic stenosis; post-partum sterilization; post-perfusion syndrome; Primary Physician Service
ppt.	*praecipitatus* (precipitate)
PPTL	post-partum tubal ligation
PPV	positive-pressure ventilation
PQ	permeability quotient; plasto-quinone
p.r.	*per rectum* (through the rectum); *pro recto* (rectal)
pr.	pair; presbyopia; prism; production; propyl
Pr	Praseodymium
P&R	pulse and respiration
PR	pain reaction; partial remission; partial response; pathology report; pelvic rock; peripheral resistance; per rectum; picture-recording; pre-record; pre-recorded; progesterone receptor; protein; public relation; pulse rate; *punctum remotum*
p.r.a.	*pro ratione aetatis* (in proportion to age)
PRA	plasma renin activity; progesterone receptor assay
PRBC	packed red blood cells
PRC	packed red cells; plasma renin concentration
PRCA	pure red cell aplasia
PRD	post-radiation dysplasia; product; production
Pred.	Prednisone
preg.	pregnant
PreMACE	Prednisone, Methotrexate, Adriamycin, Cytoxan, Etoposide
pre-op.	pre-operation; pre-operative
prep.	preparation; prepare
prep'd	prepared
PRERLA	Pupils Round, Equal, Reactive to Light and Accommodation
PRF	prolactin releasing factor
PRFM	prolonged-rupture of a fetal membrane
PRH	prolactin-releasing hormone
PRIST	paper radio-immuno-sorbent test
prl.	prolactin
PRM	phospho-ribo-mutase; premature rupture of membranes

p.r.n.	*pro re nata* (as occasion arises; as needed)
PRNT	plaque reduction neutralization test
PRO	Peer Review Organization; professional; prothrombin
prob.	probability; probable; problem
Proc.	Procarbazine; procedure; proceed; proceedings; process
Proc AACR	Proceedings — American Association for Cancer Research
Proc ASCO	Proceedings — American Society of Clinical Oncology
procto.	proctoscopy
prof.	profession; professor
prog.	prognosis; program (programme); progress; progressive
PROM	passive range of motion; premature rupture of membrane; Programmable Read Only Memory; prolonged rupture of membrane
ProMACE	Procarbazine, Methotrexate, Adriamycin, Cytoxan, Etoposide
pro rect.	*pro recto* (rectal)
PROS	professionals
prot.	protein; protocol
Pro. time	prothrombin time
prov.	provision; provisional
PRP	phosphosyl-ribitol-phosphate; pityriasis rubra pilaris; platelet-rich plasma; progesterone receptor protein
PRPC	pan-retinal photo-coagulation
PRPP	phospho-ribosyl-pyro-phosphate
PRRE	pupils round, regular, equal
PRT	phospho-ribosyl-transferase
PRTA	proximal renal tubular acidosis
PRU	peripheral resistance unit
PRV	pseudo-rabies virus
p.s.	per second; pico-second; *post scriptum* (post-script)
ps	pico-second
Ps	*Pseudomonas*
P&S	permanent and stationary
PS	pathological stage; pathological staging; phosphatidyl-serine; plastic surgery; population sample; post-script; prescription; primary stage; pulmonary stenosis; pyloric stenosis
PSA	platelet-specific antibody; polyethylene sulfonic acid; prostate-specific antigen
PSCC	posterior sub-capsular cataract
PSCT	peripheral stem cell transplantation

PSD	pelvic sidewall dissection; peptone, starch, dextrose
psec	pico-second
psf	pounds per square foot
PSG	peak systolic gallop; poly-sono-gram; pre-systolic gallop
PSGN	post-streptococcal glomerulo-nephritis
psi	para-psychological; pounds per square inch; psychological
PSIFT	platelet suspension immuno-fluorescence test
PSIS	posterior superior iliac spine
PSM	pan-systolic murmur; pre-systolic murmur
PSMF	protein-supplemented modified fast
PSNP	progressive supra-nuclear palsy
PSP	periodic short pulse; phenol-sulfon-phthalein
PSRO	Professional Standards Review Organization
PSS	progressive systemic sclerosis
PST	Pacific Standard Time; Penicillin, Streptomycin, Tetracycline
PST-PS	post-surgical treatment — pathological staging
PSV	pressure support ventilation
PSVTc	paroxysmal supra-ventricular tachy-cardia
PSWD	pelvic side-wall dissection
pt.	part; patient; *perstetur* (let it be continued); pint (from French: pinte); point; port
Pt	Platinum
PT	para-thormone; para-thyroid; para-tuberculosis; para-typhoid; part-time; pathological treatment; patient; photo-toxicity; Physical Therapist; physical therapy; Platinol; platinum; posterior tibial; proficiency testing; prothrombin time
PTA	persistent truncus arteriosus; phospho-tungstic acid; plasma thromboplastin antecedent; post-traumatic amnesia; post-traumatic arthritis; prior to admission
PTAHt	phospho-tungstic acid hema-toxylin
PTAP	percutaneous transluminal angio-plasty
PTB	patellar tendon bearing; prior to birth; pulmonary tuberculosis
PTC	paroxysmal tachy-cardia; percutaneous transhepatic cholangiography; phenyl-thio-carbamide; plasma thromboplastin component
PTCA	percutaneous transluminal coronary angioplasty
PTCAP	percutaneous transluminal coronary angio-plasty
PTCG	percutaneous transhepatic cholangio-graphy

PTD	permanent and total disability
PTE	proximal tibial epiphysis; pulmonary thrombo-embolism
PTED	pulmonary thrombo-embolic disease
PTFE	poly-tetra-fluoro-ethylene (Fluon; Fluoroflex; Teflon)
PT-FU	Platinol, Fluorouracil
PTH	para-thyroid hormone; post-transfusional hepatitis
PTHB	percutaneous trans-hepatic biopsy
PTHBD	percutaneous trans-hepatic biliary drainage
PTHS	para-thyroid hormone secretion
PTHSE	percutaneous trans-hepatic stone extraction
PTHSI	percutaneous transhepatic stent insertion
PTI	persistent tolerant infection
PTLF	passive transferable lethal factor
PTMA	phenyl-tri-methyl-ammonium
PTMV	percutaneous transvenous mitral valvotomy
p.t.o.	please turn over
PTP	post-tetanic potentiation; post-transfusion purpura
PTPT	partial thrombo-plastin time
PTR	patient to return; phosphorous tubular reabsorption
PTS	post-transfusion syndrome; post-traumatic stress
PTSA	para-toluene-sulfonic acid
PTT	pro-thrombin time
PTT/PTPT	pro-thrombin time / partial thrombo-plastin time (ratio)
PTU	propyl-thio-uracil
PTy	para-thyroidectomy
PTZ	pentylene-tetra-zol
Pu	Plutonium
PU	peptic ulcer; pregnancy urine
PUCBS	percutaneous umbilical cord blood sampling
PUD	peptic ulcer disease
PUE	pyrexia of unknown etiology
PUF	pure ultra-filtration
PUFA	poly-unsaturated fatty acid
pulm.	*pulmentum* (gruel); pulmonary
pulv.	*pulvieres* (powders); *pulvis* (powder)
PUO	pyrexia of unknown origin
PUPPP	pruritic urticarial papules and plaques of pregnancy
PUS	poison by unknown substance
PUVA	psoralen and ultra-violet A
p.v.	*partitis vicibus* (in divided dose); *per vaginam* (through the vagina); polycythemia vera

P&V	pyloroplasty and vagotomy
P/V	perfusion / ventilation
PV	peak voltage; peripheral vascular; peripheral vein; plasma volume; poly-vinyl; polycythemia vera; portal vein; pressure velocity; pulmonic valve
PVA	poly-vinyl acetate; poly-vinyl alcohol
PVB	Platinol, Velban, Bleomycin; premature ventricular beat
PVC	poly-vinyl-chloride; premature ventricular complex; premature ventricular contraction; pulmonary venous congestion
PVD	peripheral vascular disease; pulmonary vascular disease
PVE	prosthetic valve endocarditis
PVEC	prosthetic valve endo-carditis
PVHt	pulmonary venous hyper-tension
PVI	peripheral vascular insufficiency
PVM	peak voltage measurement; pneumonia virus of mice
P-VM26	Platinol, Teniposide
PVOD	peripheral vascular occlusive disease; pulmonary venous obstructive disease
PVOM	pyogenic vertebral osteo-myelitis
PVp	Platinol, Etoposide
PVP	penicillin V potassium; peripheral vein plasma; peripheral venous pressure; poly-vinyl-pyrrolidone; portal venous pressure; pulmonary venous pressure
PVP-I	poly-vinyl-pyrrolidone and iodine (povidone and iodine)
PVp-XRT	Platinol, Etoposide — Radiation Therapy
PVR	peripheral vascular resistance; pulmonary vascular resistance
PVS	premature ventricular systole
PVT	portal vein thrombosis; pressure, volume, temperature; private
PVTc	paroxysmal ventricular tachy-cardia
PW	penetrating water; plain water; plantar wart; poisoned water; posterior wall; pulse wave; pure water; purified water
PWA	person with AIDS
PWB	partial weight bearing
PWI	posterior wall infarct
PWM	port-wine mark (nevus; port-wine stain)
PWP	pulmonary wedge pressure
PWR	power
PWS	port-wine stain (nevus; port-wine mark)

pwt	penny-weight
Px	pneumothorax
PX	physical examination; please exchange; post exchange
PXE	pseudo-xanthoma elasticum
pxm.	pyrido-xa-mine
Pyr.	pyridine
PZ	pancreo-zymin; peripheral zone
PZA	pyra-zin-amide
PZCCK	pancreo-zymin-chole-cysto-kinin
PZCK	pancreo-zymin-cholecysto-kinin
PZI	protamine zinc insulin
PZP	pregnancy zone protein

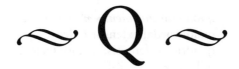

$\dot{Q}$	distribution (perfusion); rate of blood flow
$\dot{Q}_s$	physiological shunt
$\dot{Q}_s/\dot{Q}_T$	intrapulmonary shunt fraction
$\dot{Q}_T$	cardiac output
$\dot{Q}_{VA}/\dot{Q}_T$	venous admixture
q.	electric charge quantity; quantum; *quaque* (each; every); quart
q	long arm of chromosome; electric charge quantity; quantity of heat
Q	heat; quaalude (Dormutil; Methaqualone; Soverin); quadrupedal; quality; quantity; quarantine; quartz; query; question; quittor (quitter); symbol for Coulomb; ubiquinones
Q_{10}	temperature coefficient
Q-275	ubiquinones
QA	qualitative analysis; quality assurance
QAB	quaternary ammonium bases
QAC	quaternary ammonium compound
QALY	quality-adjusted life year
QALYs	quality-adjusted life years
q.a.m.	every morning
Q-band.	quinacrine-banding
QC	quality control
QCO_2	number of microliters (microlitres) of carbon dioxide
QC-PCR	competitive polymerase-chain reaction
QCT	Quantitative Computed Tomography
q.d.	*quaque die* (every day)
q. day	every day
QDHC	quinine di-hydro-chloride
q.d.s.	*quater die sumendum* (to be taken four times a day)
q.e.	*quod est* (which is)
q.e.d.	*quod erat demonstrandum* (which was to be demonstrated)
q.e.f.	*quod erat faciendum* (which was to be done)

q.e.i.	*quod erat inveniendum* (which was to be found out)
QER	quadrupedal extensor reflex
QF	quadriceps femoris; quality factor; query fever (nine-mile fever); quick-firing
q. fever	quarten fever (quartan malaria); quotidian fever
q.h.	*quaque hora* (every hour)
q.2h.	*quaque secunda hora* (every second hour)
q.3h.	*quaque tertia hora* (every third hour)
q.4h.	*quaque quarta hora* (every fourth hour)
QHC	quinacrine hydro-chloride
q.h.s.	*quaque hora somni* (each bed-time)
QICA	Quantitative Inhalation Challenge Apparatus
q.i.d.	*quater in die* (four times a day)
q.l.	*quantum libet* (as much as is desired)
q.m.	*quaque mane* (every morning); *quaque matin* (every morning)
QM	quartan malaria (quartan fever)
QMB	Qualified Medicare Beneficiary
q. month	every month
QMS	Qualified Medical Student
q.m.t.	quantitative muscle testing
QMT	quantitative muscle testing
q.n.	*quaque nocte* (every night); *quaque nox* (every night)
q.n.s.	quantity not sufficient
QO_2	number of microliters (microlitres) of oxygen consumption
q.o.d.	*every other day*
q.o.l.	quality of life
q.o.s.	*quoties opus sit* (as often as necessary)
q.p.	*quantum placet* (as much as you please); *quantum placetat* (as much as you please; as you will)
QP	quadriceps femoris
q.p.m.	every afternoon; every evening
qq.	*quaque* (each; every); question
QqD	Quinquaud's Disease
Qq-disease	Quinquaud's disease
q.q.h.	*quaque quarta hora* (every fourth hour)
qq. hor.	*quaque hora* (every hour)
qqv	*quae vide* (which see...used in plural form)
q.r.	*quantum rectum* (the quantity is correct)
qr.	quarter
QRS	Q wave, R wave, S wave
QRST	Q wave, R wave, S wave, T wave

q.s.	quantity sufficient; *quantum sufficiat* (as much as will suffice; enough); *quantum satis* (sufficient quantity); *quantum sufficit* (as much as necessary)
QS	Queckenstedt's sign; Quevenne scale; quinidine sulfate
qt.	quantity; *quartina* (quart)
QT	quinine tannate
qtr.	quarter
qts.	quarters; quarts
QTT-fev.	Queensland tick typhus fever
qtts.	quantities
qty.	quantity
qu.	question
quad.	quadriceps; quadriplegic; quadruped; quadruplet
quadrup.	*quadruplicato* (four times as much)
quat.	*quattour* (four)
ques.	question
QUH	quinine and urea hydrochloride
quin.	*quinque* (five)
quot.	*quatidie* (daily; every day)
q.v.	*quantum vis* (as much as you wish; which see); *quantum voleris* (as much as you wish; which see)
q. 2wk	every 2 weeks
q. 4wk	every 4 weeks

~ R ~

r	correlation coefficient; radius distance; *remotum* (far); resistance of drug; röntgen (roentgen); *ruber* (red)
R	race; radiation; radio; radius; Rankine; rate; ratio; reactance; reaction; reactive; recovery; rectal; red; reference; region; register; registered; regression; relation; relative; relaxed; remark; renal; repeat; report; resident; residual tumor; residual; resistance; resistance; respiration; rest; reverse; rhythm; right; room; root; rotary; rough; round; rub; rupture; Russia; Russian
R0	residual tumor — none
R1	residual tumor — microscopic
R2	residual tumor — macroscopic
R_A	airway resistance
R_e	Reynold's number
R_p	pulmonary resistance
R_x	*recipe* (dispense: used at the beginning of a prescription)
Ra	Radium
RA	rectal alimentation; rectal anesthesia; refractory anemia; renal artery; repeat action; rheumatoid arthritis; right anterior right arm; right atrial; right atrium; right auricle
RAAg	rheumatoid arthritis agglutination
RAANA	rheumatoid arthritis-associated nuclear antigen
RAAPI	resting ankle arm pressure index
RAC	Remak's axis cylinder; rheumatoid arthritis cell
RACAD	rapid acquisition computed axial tomography
rad.	radial; radian; radiation; radium; radius; *radix* (root)
RAD	radian; right axis deviation; radiation absorbed dose; reactive airway disease; right anterior descending
RADAR	radio detecting and ranging
RADIAC	radio-active detection, identification and countermeasures
RADTS	rabbit anti-dog thymus serum
RAE	right atrial enlargement
RAF	rheumatoid arthritis factor

RAG	radio-autograph; reticular apparatus of Golgi
RAH	regressing atypical histiocytosis; right atrial hypertrophy
RAI	radio-active iodine
RAIHSA	radio-active iodinated human serum albumin
RAISA	radio-active iodinated serum albumin
RAIU	radio-active iodine uptake
RAM	Random Access Memory; random alternating movements; rapid alternating movements
RAM-1	rectus abdominis muscle (flap) — unilateral
RAM-2	rectus abdominis muscle (flap) — bilateral
R.A.M.C.	Royal Army Medical Corps
RAMF	rectus abdominis myocutaneous flap
RAMF-1	rectus abdominis muscle flap — unilateral
RAMF-2	rectus abdominis muscle flap — bilateral
RAMP	Rifamycin-AMP (Rifampicin; Rifampin; Riforal)
RAMT	rabbit anti-mouse thymocyte
RAO	right anterior oblique
RAP	rheumatoid arthritis precipitation; right atrial pressure
RAPS	Rapid Acute Physiology Score
RARLS	rabbit anti-rat lymphocyte serum
ras.	*rasrae* (fillings; scrapings)
RAS	renal artery stenosis; reticular-activating system
RAST	radio-allergo-sorbent test; rheumatoid arthritis slide test
RAT	radial aplasia thrombocytopenia
RATG	rabbit anti-thymocyte globulin
RaTx	radiation therapy
RAU	radio-active uptake
RAV	Rous-associated virus
RAW	resistance of air-way
RAWEBIT	refractory anemia with excess blasts in transformation
Rb	Rubidium
RB	rachitic beads; red blindness; respiratory bronchiole; Russell bodies; Russian bath
RBA	regional block anesthesia; right brachial artery; rose bengal antigen
RBB	retro-bulbar block; right bundle branch
RBBB	right bundle branch block
RBC	red blood cell; red blood count
RBC/hpf	red blood cell per high power field
RBC-ITO	red blood cell iron turn-over
RBCM	red blood cell mass
RBCV	red blood cell volume

RBD	rheumatic brain disease
RBE	relative biological effectiveness
RBER	relative biological effectiveness of radiation
RBF	renal blood flow
RBL	Reid's base line
RBM	rachial-bumini-meter; rachial-bumini-metry
RBP	retinal-binding protein
RBS	random blood sugar
RBV	right brachial vein
R.C.	Red Cross; Roman Catholic
RC	radical cystectomy; reticuloendothelial cell; retinal correspondence; retinitis circinata; retinitis circumpapillaris; rhinitis caseosa; rib cage; rima cornealis; rough colony
RCA	right coronary artery
RCBF	regional cerebral blood flow
RCBV	regional cerebral blood volume
RCC	red cell count; renal cell carcinoma
RCCA	right common carotid artery
RCD	relative cardiac dullness
RCDW	red cell diameter width; red cell distribution width
RCF	red cell folate; relative centrifugal force; root canal filling
RCFR	red cell flow rate
RCG	retrograde cysto-gram
RCIA	red cell immune adherence
RCIARF	radio contrast-induced acute renal failure
RCITOR	red cell iron turn-over rate
RCM	red cell mass; right costal margin; Royal College of Midwives
RCN	Royal College of Nursing
RCO	aliphatic acyl radical
RCOG	Royal College of Obstetricians and Gynaecologists
RCP	Royal College of Physician
RCPP	regional cerebral perfusion pressure
RCPS	Royal College of Physicians and Surgeons
RCR	respiratory control ratio
RCS	reticulum cell sarcoma; Royal College of Surgeons
RCT	recalcified clotting time; renal clearance test; root canal treatment
RCU	red cell utilization
RCV	red cell volume
RCVS	Royal College of Veterinary Surgeons

RCWI	right cardiac work index
R&D	research and development
RD	Ranikhet disease; Raynaud's disease; reaction of generation; reading disorders; Reclus' disease; reduction diet; reduction division; reference delusion; renal decortication; resistance determinant; retarded depression; retinal detachment; right deltoid; road; rod; round
RDA	recommended daily allowance; recommended dietary allowance; right dorso-anterior (fetus position)
RDCSRV	Rheus diploid cell strain rabies vaccine
RDD	random digit dial
RDE	receptor-destroying enzyme
RDFS	ratio of decayed and filled surface
R.D.H.	Registered Dental Hygienist
RDI	relative dose intensity; respiratory disturbance index; rupture delivery interval
rDNA	ribosomal deoxy-ribo-nucleic acid
RDP	right dorso-posterior (fetus position)
RDR	relative dose response
RDS	respiratory distress syndrome
RDSN	respiratory distress syndrome of the newborn
Re	Rhenium
RE	radiation emanation; radium emanation; random error; rectal examination; regional enteritis; reticulo-endothelial; retinal equivalent; right ear; right eye
REA	radio-enzymatic assay; radiological emergency assistance
rec.	receive; *recens* (fresh); recipient; record; recreation; rectum
REC	receive; receiver; recommend; recommendation; record
rec'd	received
RECG	radio-electrocardiogram; radio-electro-cardiography
re-ch.	re-check
recip.	recipient
rect.	*rectificatus* (rectified); rectum
RE-DF	Rees and Ecker's diluting fluid
REE	resting energy expenditure
re-exam.	re-examination
REF	referee; reference; refuse; refused; renal erythropoietic factor
reg.	region; register; registration; regular
REG	radio-encephalo-gram; radio-encephalo-graphy
rehab.	rehabilitation

REKG	radio-electro-kardio-gram (radio-electro-cardiogram); radio-electro-kardio-graphy (radio-electro-cardio-graphy)
REL	radiation exposure limit; recommended exposure limit; relative
REM	rapid eye movement; roentgen equivalent man
REMP	roentgen equivalent man period
REMS	rapid eye movement sleep (paradoxical sleep)
ren ∠	renal angle
ren. sem.	*renovetur semel* (shall be renewed only once)
REO	respiratory and enteric orphan
REOV	respiratory and enteric orphan virus
rep.	repair; *repetatur* (let it be repeated); report; representative
REP	rapid ejection period; roentgen equivalent physical; representative
REPG	radio-electro-physiolo-graphy
rept.	*repetatur* (let it be repeated)
RER	renal excretion rate; respiratory exchange ratio; rough endoplasmic reticulum
res.	research; reserve; residence; resident; residue; resolution
RES	reticulo-endothelial system; resident
resp.	respectively; respiration; respiratory; response
ret.	retire; retreat; retrieve; return
RET	roentgen equivalent therapy
rev.	reverse; review; reviewed; revised; revision
REV	reticulo-endotheliosis virus
RF	rabbit fever; radio frequency; regurgitation factor; relative fluorescence; releasing factor; renal failure; respiratory failure; rheumatic fever; rheumatoid factor
RFA	rachitis fetalis annularis; right femoral artery; right fore-arm; right fronto-anterior (fetus position)
RFD	residue free diet; Riga-Fede's disease
RFER	radio-frequency electrophrenic respiration
RFL	right fronto-lateral (fetus position)
RFLA	rheumatoid factor-like activity
RFLP	restriction fragment length polymorphism
RFM	rachitis fetalis micromelica
RFP	rachitic flat pelvis; right fronto-posterior (fetus position)
RFPS	Royal Faculty of Physicians and Surgeons
RFS	relapse-free survival; renal function study
RFT	Reed-Frost theory; right fronto-transverse (fetus position)

RFW	rapid filling wave
RG	radio-gram; radio-grapher; radio-graphy; reflexo-graphy; retro-graphy; right gluteal
RGN	Registered General Nurse
rh	relative humidity; rheumatic; rheumatoid
Rh	Rhesus; Rhesus factor; Rhodium
RH	reactive hyperemia; relative humidity; releasing hormone; right hand; right hyperphoria
Rh⁻	Rhesus negative factor
Rh⁺	Rhesus positive factor
RhBF	Rhodium blood factor
RHBF	reactive hyperemia blood flow
RhBG	Rhodium blood group
RHD	relative hepatic dullness; rheumatic heart disease
RHEP	recombinant human erythro-poietin
RHF	right heart failure
RHG-CSF	recombinant human granulocyte colony-stimulating factor
RHL	right hepatic lobe
RHLN	right hilar lymph node
r.h.m.	roentgen-hour-meter (röntgen-hour-metre)
RHS	right hand side
RI	recession index; refractive index; regional ileitis; regular insulin; respiratory illness
RIA	radio-immuno-assay
RIC	Royal Institute of Chemistry
RICM	right inter-costal margin
RICU	Respiratory Intensive Care Unit
RID	radial immuno-diffusion; radio-immuno-detection; reciprocal inhibition and desensitization
RIDA	radial-immuno-diffusion assay
RIF	right iliac fossa
RIFA	radio-iodinated fatty acid
RIH	right inguinal hernia
RIMA	right internal mammary artery
RIND	resolving ischemic neurological deficit; reversible ischemic neurological disability
r.i.p.	*redigatur in pulverem* (let it be reduced to powder); *reductus in pulverem* (reduced to powder)
RIP	radio-immuno-precipitation; *requiescant in pace* (may they rest in peace); *requiescat in pace* (may he rest in peace); rest in peace

RIPA	radio-immuno-precipitation assay
RIPHH	Royal Institute of Public Health and Hygiene
RIPT	radio-immuno-precipitin test
RIR	right iliac region
RISA	radio-active iodinated serum albumin
RIST	radio-immuno-sorbent test
RITA	radium intra-tumoral application
RIU	radioactive iodine uptake
RK	rabbit kidney; radial keratotomy; right kidney; right knee
RKY	roentgen-kymography
R→L	right to left
R&L	right and left
RL	reflected light; reflex light; reticular layer; right leg; right line; right lower; right lung; Ringer's lactate; round ligament
RLAR	repeat low anterior resection
RLBCD	right lower border of cardiac dullness
RLC	residual lung capacity
RLE	right lower extremity
RLFP	retro-lental fibro-plasia
RLL	radio-lucent line; right lower limb; right lower lobe; right lower lung
RLM	radiation leak measurement
RLN	recurrent laryngeal nerve
RLP	radiation leukemia protection
RLQ	right lower quadrant
RLR	right lateral rectus
RLS	Ringer's lactate solution
RLV	radiation leukemia virus
rm	roentgen-meter (röntgen-metre)
RM	radical mastectomy; reference man; reference material; rheumatoid myositis; Roger murmur; room
RMA	right mento-anterior (fetus position)
RMBF	regional myocardial blood flow
RMCA	right middle cerebral artery
RMCBF	regional myo-cardial blood flow
RMK	Rhesus monkey kidney
RML	right middle lobe; right middle lung
RMM	radiculo-meningo-myelitis
RMP	resting membrane potential; right mento-posterior (fetus position)

RMQ	right middle quadrant
RMR	right medial rectus
RMRV	Rhesus monkey rota-virus
rms	root-mean-square
RMS	resident medical staff
RMSF	Rocky Mountain spotted fever
RMT	right mento-transverse (fetus position)
RMV	respiratory minute volume
Rn	Radon
R.N.	Registered Nurse
RNA	ribo-nucleic acid
RNAG	radio-nuclide angio-graphy
RNase	ribo-nucle-ase
RND	radical neck dissection; regional neck dissection; regional node dissection; round
RNE	relativity not established
RNP	ribo-nucleo-protein
RNVG	radio-nucleotide veno-graphy
R/O	ruled out; rule out
RO	red-out; relative odds; routine order
ROA	range of accommodation; received on account; right occipito-anterior (fetus position)
ROAD	reversible obstructive airways disease
ROB	riding of bones
ROD	reaction of degeneration; renal osteo-dystrophy
ROE	refraction of eye
ROHT	rat ovarian hyperemia test
ROI	reservoir of infection
ROL	right occipito-lateral (fetus position)
ROM	range of motion; Read-Only Memory; right otitis media; rupture of membrane
RON	rule of nines
ROP	raphe of penis; retinopathy of prematurity; right occipito-posterior (fetus position); rupture of perineum
ROS	review of system
ROSC	return of spontaneous circulation
ROT	raphe of tongue; remedial occupational therapy; right occipito-transverse (fetus position); rupture of tubes
ROU	retroversion of uterus; rupture of uterus
RP	reactive protein; radial pulse; rapid process; referred pain; refractive power; resting period; retrograde pyelogram

RPA	retinitis punctata albescens; reverse passive anaphylaxis; right pulmonary artery
RPB	retinal binding protein
RPC	red pulp cords
RPCF	Reiter protein complement fixation
RPCFT	Reiter protein complement fixation test
RPE	retinal pigment epithelium
RPF	renal plasma flow
RPG	retrograde pyelo-gram
RPGN	rapidly progressive glomerulo-nephritis
R.Ph.	Registered Pharmacist
RPI	reticulocytic production index
RPKT	reversed Prausnitz-Küstner test
RPL	radiological path length; retro-peritoneal lymphadenectomy
r.p.m.	revolutions per minute; rounds per minute
RPN	renal papillary necrosis; resident's progress note
RPO	right posterior oblique
RPR	rapid plasma reagin
RPRCT	rapid plasma reagin card test
RPRT	rapid plasma reagin test
r.p.s.	rounds per second
RPS	renal pressor substance; resident physician section
rpt.	repeat; report
R.P.T.	Registered Physical Therapist
RPV	right pulmonary vein
RQ	respiratory quotient
R&R	rate and rhythm; recess and resect; remove and replace; rest and recuperation
RR	reaction response; radiation response; recovery room; relative risk; renin release; respiratory rate; response rate
R.R.A.	Registered Record Administrator
RRA	radio-receptor assay
RRE	round, regular, equal
R.R.L.	Registered Record Librarian
rRNA	ribosomal ribo-nucleic acid
RRR	regular rhythm and rate; renin release rate
RRT	relative retention time
r.s.	*renovetur semel* (shall be renewed only once)
RS	railway sickness; Reiter's syndrome; respiratory syncytium; right side; Ringer's solution; Romanovsky stain; rose spots

199

RSA	reticulum cell sarcoma; right sacro-anterior (fetus position)
RSC	rested state contraction
RScA	right scapulo-anterior (fetus position)
RSCA	right sub-clavian artery
RS-cell	Reed-Sternberg cell
RScP	right scapulo-posterior (fetus position)
RSCV	right sub-clavian vein
RSD	reflex sympathetic dystrophy; relative standard deviation; residual standard deviation
RSDS	reflex sympathetic dystrophy syndrome
RSDV	respiratory sialo-dacryoadenitis virus
RSE	recurrent summer eruption (hydroa vacciniforme); reference standard endotoxin
RSI	repetitive strain injury
RSM	Royal Society of Medicine
RSNA	Radiological Society of North America
RSP	right sacro-posterior (fetus position)
RSR	regular sinus rhythm
RST	radio-sensitivity test; right sacro-transverse (fetus position)
RSTL	relaxed skin tension lines
RSTMH	Royal Society of Tropical Medicine and Hygiene
RSV	respiratory syncytial virus; Rous sarcoma virus
R.S.V.P.	please reply (French: répondez s'il vous plaît)
RSWC	right side up with care
R.T.	Registered Technologist
RT	radiation therapy; radio-therapy; radium therapy; reaction time; reading test; respiratory therapy; right; right thigh; room temperature
RTA	renal tubular acidosis
RTAS	rat thymus anti-serum
RTBC	Russian tick-borne complex (encephalitides)
RTC	return to clinic
RTD	returned; resubmission turnaround document; resubmission turnaround documents; routine test dilution
RTF	resistance transfer factor; respiratory tract fluid
RT+FU	radiation therapy and Fluorouracil
RTH	return to hospital
RTOG	Radiation Therapy Oncology Group
RT-PA	recombinant tissue plasminogen activator

RTS	request to send
RT3U	resin triiodothyronine uptake
RTx	radiation therapy
ru	radiation unit
Ru	Ruthenium
RU	rat unit; residual urine; resistance unit; rodent ulcer; roentgen unit (röntgen unit)
RU486	abortifacient pill
rub.	*ruber* (red)
RUE	right upper extremity
RUG	retrograde uretero-gram
RUL	right upper limb; right upper lobe; right upper lung
RUOQ	right upper outer quadrant
rup'd	ruptured
rupt.	rupture; ruptured
RUQ	right upper quadrant
RUR	resin uptake ratio
RURTI	recurrent upper respiratory tract infection
RUS	Russia; Russian
RV	rabies vaccine; rat virus; recreational vehicle; residual volume; respiratory volume; return visit; right ventricle; rima vocalis; rubella virus
RVA	right ventricular apex
RVAD	right ventricular assist device
RVB	red venous blood
RVD	relative vertebral density; right ventricular dimension
RVDV	right ventricular diastolic volume
RVE	right ventricular enlargement
RVEDP	right ventricular end-diastolic pressure
RVEDV	right ventricular end-diastolic volume
RVEF	right ventricular ejection fraction
RVEP	right ventricular ejection period
RVESP	right ventricular end-systolic pressure
RVESV	right ventricular end-systolic volume
RVET	right ventricular ejection time
RVH	reno-vascular hypertension; right ventricular hypertrophy
RVID	right ventricular internal dimension
RVO	relaxed vaginal outlet
RVOA	right ventricular over-activity
RVOT	right ventricular outflow tract
RVPP	right ventricular pre-ejection period
RVR	renal vascular resistance

RVRA	renal vein renin activity; renal venous renin assay
RVRC	renal vein renin concentration
RVS	relative value studies
RVSV	right ventricular stroke volume
RVSWI	right ventricular stroke work index
RVT	renal vein thrombosis
RV/TLC	residual volume / total lung capacity (ratio)
RVU	relative value unit
RVVL	rubella virus vaccine live
RW	rag-weed; reference woman; rose water
RWC	resting wandering cell
RWO	Risky work-out
RX	*recipe* (take); therapy; treatment; medication; drug
ryt.	rytidosis

∼ S ∼

$\bar{s}$	*sine* (without)
$\hat{S}$	spatial vector in electro-cardiology
s.	*sans* (without); *semis* (half); *signa* (mark; sign, write); *sinister* (left)
S	entropy; Salmonella; salt; Schistosoma; school; second; seconds; section; serum; shock; short; sick; single; sister; size; skin; small; smooth; soluble; son; sone; sound; south; sphere; Spirillum; standard; Staphylococcus; stomach; Streptococcus; Streptozocin; substrate; sulfur; surgery; Svedberg
S_1	first heart sound; primary syphilis
S_2	second heart sound; secondary syphilis
S_{2p}	pulmonic valve closure
S_3	third heart sound; tertiary syphilis; ventricular gallop
S_4	atrial gallop; fourth heart sound
S_f	Svedberg flotation unit
S_F	Svedberg sedimentation unit
S1	first sacral vertebra (first sacral nerve)
S2	second sacral vertebra (second sacral nerve)
S6	ribosomal protein
S-30	late latent syphilis
S-40	late syphilis
s.a.	*secundum artem* (according to art; by skill)
Sa.	Samarium; Saturday
SA	saccharum album; salicylic acid; Saturday; sclerotic acid; secondary amenorrhea; secondary anemia; serum albumin; sino-atrial; sino-auricular; sinus arrest; sinus arrhythmia; sleep apnea; sleeping area; soda ash (sodium-carbonate); spasmus agitans; surface area; sustained action
SAA	serum amyloid A; severe aplastic anemia; Stokes-Adams attack
SAB	significant asymptomatic bacteriuria; sino-atrial block; spontaneous abortion; sub-arachnoid block
SAC	short arm cast; spinal-accessory chain

SACE	serum angiotensin converting enzyme
SACH	single axis cushioned-heel; solid ankle cushioned-heel
SACT	sino-atrial conduction time
SAD	seasonal affective disorder; Stokes-Adams disease
SAE	sea algae extraction
SAECG	signal-averaged electro-cardio-gram
SAF	Saint Anthony's fire; serum accelerator factor
SAGES	Society of American Gastrointestinal Endoscopic Surgeons
SAH	sub-arachnoid hemorrhage
SAIDS	simian-acquired immune deficiency syndrome
SAIMR	South African Institute for Medical Research
s.a.l.	*secundum artis leges* (according to the rules of art)
sal.	salicylate; salimeter; saline; saliva; salivation
SAM	smoking-attributable mortality; surface active material; systolic anterior motion
SAMMEL	smoking-attributable mortality, morbidity, and economic loss
SAN	sino-atrial node
SANC	short arm navicular cast
SAO	stimulated acid output
SAO_2	arterial oxygen percent saturation
SAP	serum alkaline phosphatase; systemic arterial pressure
SAPS	Simplified Acute Physiology Score
SART	sino-atrial recovery time
SAS	short-arm splint; sleep apnea syndrome; Statistical Analysis System; Stokes-Adams syndrome
SASPE	sub-acute sclerosing pan-encephalitis
sat.	saturate; saturation; *saturatus* (saturated)
Sat.	Saturday
SAT	Saturday; Scholastic Aptitude Test; Senior Apperception Test
sat. sol.	saturated solution
SAVE	survival and ventricular enlargement
Sb	*Stibium* (antimony)
SB	sacral bone; saddle block; serum bilirubin; single breath; sitz bath (hip bath); sleeping bag; small bowel; snow blindness; sternal border; still-birth
$SbCl_3$	antimony-trichloride
SB-CPAP	spontaneous breathing with continuous positive airway pressure
SBD_{CO}	single breath diffusing capacity for carbon monoxide
SBE	sea-bather's eruption; subacute bacterial endocarditis

SBF	splanchnic blood flow
SBFT	small bowel follow-through (X-ray study)
SBI	serious bacterial infection
SBN	single breath nitrogen (test)
SBO	small bowel obstruction
Sb_2O_3	antimony-trioxide
Sb_2O_5	antimony-pentoxide
SBOM	soy-bean oil meal
SBP	spontaneous bacterial peritonitis; systemic blood pressure; systolic blood pressure
SBRN	sensory branch of radial nerve
Sb_2S_3	antimony-trisulfide
SBT	serum bacterial titer
SBTI	soy-bean trypsin inhibitor
SB tube	Sengstaken-Blackmore tube
SBV	single binocular vision
SBW	spectral band-width
s̄c	without correction (eye-glasses)
s̄ / c	without correction (eye-glasses)
s.c.	*sub cutis* (sub-cutaneously)
Sc	Scandium
S&C	sclerae and conjunctivae
SC	saccharum canadense (maple sugar); saccharum candidum (rock candy); sacral canal; sacro-coccygeal; salaam convulsion; secretory component; self-care; self-cueing; serum chemistry; sickle cell; simian crease; sterno-clavicular; sub-clavian; subcutaneous
SCA	sickle cell anemia; *Staphylococcus cereus aureus*
SCAB	Streptozotocin, CCNU, Adriamycin, Bleomycin
SCAG	selective coronary angiogram
scat.	*scatula* (box)
SCAT	sheep cell agglutination test; sickle cell anemia test
scat. orig.	*scatula originalis* (original package)
SCC	small cell carcinoma; squamous cell cancer; squamous cell carcinoma
SCCB	small cell carcinoma of the bone
SCCHN	squamous cell carcinoma of head and neck
SCCM	Society of Critical Care Medicine
SCCV	squamous cell carcinoma of vulva
Sc.D.	Doctor of Science
SCD	sick cell disease; subacute combined degeneration; sudden cardiac death; sudden coronary death
ScDA	scapulo-dextra anterior (fetus position)

SC disease	sickle cell disease; sickle cell-hemolglobin C disease
ScDP	scapulo-dextra posterior (fetus position)
SCDT	solid carbon dioxide therapy
SCE	secretory carcinoma of endometrium
SCF	*Staphylococcus cereus flavus*
SCFE	slipped capital femoral epiphysis
SCG	serum chemistry graft; sodium-cromoglycate
SCI	science; scientific; spinal cord injury
SCID	severe combined immune deficiency
SCIDD	severe combined immune deficiency disorder
SCIPP	sacro-coccygeal to inferior pubic point
SCJ	squamo-columnar junction
SCK	serum creatine kinase
SCL	soft contact lens
ScLA	scapulo-laeva anterior (fetus position)
SCLC	small cell lung cancer
ScLP	scapulo-laeva posterior (fetus position)
SCM	Society of Computer Medicine; sterno-cleido-mastoid
SCN	seventh cranial nerve; sixth cranial nerve; Thio-cya-nate
Scop.	Scopolamine (Hyoscine)
SCOP	specialized center of research
SCP	single cell protein
SCPK	serum creatine phospho-kinase
SCR	silicon-controlled rectifier
SCT	sex chromatin test; staphylococcal clumping test
sctd.	scattered
SCU	special care unit
SCUBA	self-contained underwater breathing apparatus
SCUF	slow continuous ultra-filtration
s. cut.	*sub cutis* (sub-cutaneously)
SCV	sub-clavian vein
SCV-CPR	simultaneous compression-ventilation cardio-pulmo-nary resuscitation
S/D	systolic / diastolic (ratio)
SD	salt diet; septal defect; serologically defined; serum defect; shoulder disarticulation; Sippy diet; skin dose; soft diet; spontaneous delivery; stable disease; standard deviation; state disability; strepto-dornase; sudden death
SDA	sacro-dextra anterior (fetus position); serologically defined antigen; specific dynamic action
S-D curve	strength-duration curve
SDD	sterile dry dressing

SDE	specific dynamic effect; standard dose epinephrine
SDH	serine de-hydrase; sorbitol de-hydrogenase; sub-dural hematoma; succinate de-hydrogenase
SDI	standard deviation index; standard deviation interval
SDM	standard deviation of the mean
SDP	sacro-dextra posterior (fetus position); sulfur-dioxide poisoning
SDR	surgical dressing room
SDS	sodium-dodecyl-sulfate; sudden death syndrome
SDS-PAGE	sodium-dodecyl-sulfate poly-acrylamide gel electrophoresis
SDT	sacro-dextra transversa (fetus position)
Se	Selenium; September
SE	saline enema; *Salmonella enteritidis*; self-examination; side effect; side effects; special examination; sphenoethmoidal suture; standard error; status epilepticus; systematic error
sec.	second; secondary; seconds
sec. a.	*secundum artem* (according to art; by skill)
secs.	seconds
sed.	sedimentation
SED	skin erythema dose; spondylo-epiphyseal dysplasia
sed. rate	sedimentation rate (blood)
SEER	Surveillance, Epidemiology, End Result
seg.	segment; segmentation; segmentectomy; segregation
SEG	segmentectomy; sono-encephalo-gram
segs.	segmental neutrophils
sem.	seminar
SEM	scanning electron microscope; seminar; standard error of the mean; systolic ejection murmur
SEMI	*semi* (half); sub-endocardial myocardial infarction
semih.	*semihora* (half an hour)
SEO	severe external otitis
Sep.	separate; separated; September; septum
SEP	sensory evoked potential; September; systolic ejection period
sepn.	separation
Sept.	*septem* (seven); September
seq.	*sequela* (that which follows); sequential; sequestrum
ser.	serial; series; serine; serious; service
SER	sensory evoked response; supination external rotation; systolic ejection rate
serv.	*serva* (preserve); service

SES	socio-economic status; suds enema soap
sesq.	*sesquihora* (an hour and a half)
SET	systolic ejection time
Sf	Svedberg flotation unit
SF	scarlet fever; serum-fast; spinal fluid; spotted fever; synovial fluid
SFA	superficial femoral artery
s.f.c.	*sub finem coctionis* (towards the end of boiling)
SFC	spinal fluid count
SFD	salt-free diet; silver fork deformity; small-for-date (infant)
SFE	sun-flower eyes
SFEMG	single fiber electro-myo-graphy
SFM	sustentacular fibers of Müller
SFP	sodium-fluoride poisoning; spinal fluid pressure
SFW	slow-filling wave
s.g.	specific gravity
SG	saccharo-galactorrhea; security guard; serum globulin; skin graft; sun-glass; sun-glasses
SGA	small for gestational age
s.gl.	without correction; without glasses
SGOT	serum glutamic oxaloacetic transaminase (AST)
SGP	serine-glycero-phosphatide
SGPT	serum glutamic pyruvic transaminase (ALT)
SGS	silkworm gut suture
SGV	salivary gland virus
s.h.	*semihora* (half an hour)
sh.	share; shoulder
S&H	speech and hearing
SH	serum hepatitis; sex hormone; sinus histiocytosis; social history; somatotropin hormone; sulf-hydryl; surgical history
ShA	shoulder amputation
SHb	sulf-hemoglobin
SHBD	serum hydroxy-butyrate dehydrogenase
SHBG	sex hormone-binding globulin
SHEP	systolic hypertension in elderly program
SHG	synthetic human gastrin
SHOA	secondary hypertrophic osteo-arthropathy
SHP	sodium hydroxide poisoning
SHT	steroid hormone therapy
Si	Silicon

S&I	suction and irrigation
SI	International Systems (French: Système International); sacral ilia; sacral index; saturation index; self-inflicted; seriously ill; serum iron; soluble insulin; stimulation index; stroke index
SIADH	syndrome of inappropriate anti-diuretic hormone
sib.	sibling
sic.	*siccus* (dried)
SIC	Setchenov's inhibitory centers
SICD	serum iso-citric dehydrogenase
SICT	selective intra-coronary thrombolysis
SICU	Surgical Intensive Care Unit
s.i.d.	*semel in die* (once a day)
SID	source image distance; sudden infant death
SIDS	sudden infant death syndrome
SIDV	simian immune deficiency virus
SIECUS	Sex Information and Education Council of the United States
sig.	sigmoid; sigmoidoscopy; *signa* (label; write); signal; signature; *signetur* (let it be written)
SIg	surface immuno-globulin
SIJ	sacro-iliac joint
sim.	*simul* (at once; at the same time)
SIMM	Single In-Line Memory Module
simul	*simul* (at once; at the same time)
SIMV	synchronized intermittent mandatory ventilation
SIN	squamous intraepithelial neoplasia
sing.	*singulorum* (of each)
SiO$_2$	silicon-dioxide
SIOP	International Society of Pediatric Oncologists
SIP	sickness impact profile
SIRS	soluble immune response suppressor
SIRT	simultaneous iterative reconstruction technique
SISI	short increment sensitivity index
SIU	International Systems of (Metric) Units (French: Système International d'Unités)
SIV	situs inversus viscerum
SIW	self-inflicted wound
SK	sclerosing keratitis; seborrheic keratosis; skin; strepto-kinase; syncytial knot; syphilitic kidney
SK-SD	streptokinase — streptodornase
s.l.	*sequenti luce* (the following day)

sl.	slight; slightly; slim; slope; slow
SL	saccharum lactis (lactose; sugar of milk); sensational level; serious list; straight line; strepto-lysin; sub-lingual
SLA	sacro-laeva anterior (fetus position); slide latex agglutination; swine lymphocyte antigen
SLAC	scaphoid lunate advanced-collapse
SLB	short leg brace
SLC	short leg cast
SLDH	serum lactic de-hydrogenase
SLDR	sub-lethal damage repair
SLE	Saint Louis encephalitis; systemic lupus erythematosus
SLEV	Saint Louis encephalitis virus
SLH	Starling's law of heart; stella lentis hyaloidea
SLI	splenic localization index; Starling's law of intestine; stella lentis iridica
SLKC	superior limbic kerato-conjunctivitis
SLL	*stria longitudinalis lateralis*
SLN	superior laryngeal nerve
SL-O	strepto-lysin O
SLP	sacro-laeva posterior (fetus position); sex limited protein
SLR	straight leg raising; Streptococcus lactis R
SLRT	straight leg raising test
SLS	short-leg splint; superior longitudinal sinus
slt.	slight; salt
SLT	sacro-laeva transverse (fetus position)
SLWC	short leg walking cast
sm.	small
Sm	Samarium
S.M.	*Scientiae Magister* (Master of Science)
SM	Saccharomyces; slow motion; Strepto-mycin; sub-mucous; suction method; systolic mean; systolic murmur
SMA	sequential multiple analysis; sequential multiple analyzer; smooth muscle antibody; superior mesenteric artery; supplementary motor area
SMA-6	sequential multiple analysis — 6 different serum tests
SMA-12	sequential multiple analysis — 12 channel biochemical profile
SMA-20	sequential multiple analysis — 20 chemical constituents tests
SMA-60	sequential multiple analysis — 60 chemical constituents tests
SMAC	Sequential Multiple Analyzer Computer

SMAF	specific macrophage arming-actor
SMAR	Schafer's method of artificial respiration
SMAS	superficial muscular aponeurotic system
SMAST	Short Michigan Alcoholism Screening Test
SMBV	suckling mouse brain vaccine
SMC	seleno-methylnor-cholesterol
SMD	Strümpell-Marie disease; senile macular degeneration
SMF	Streptozocin, Mitomycin, Fluorouracil
SMI	sodium-morrhuate injection
SML	superior malleolar ligament
SMO	Senior Medical Officer
SMON	subacute myelo-optic neuropathy
SMOTTA	synthetic medium old tuberculin trichloroacetic acid
SMP	simultaneous macular perception; slow moving protease; Sunday morning paralysis
smr.	smear
SMR	somnolent metabolic rate; standard morbidity ratio; standard mortality ratio; sub-mucous resection
SMRR	sub-mucous resection and rhinoplasty
SMS	soft medicinal soap; stiff man syndrome
SMV	sub-mento-vertex
SMX	sulfa-metho-xazole
s.n.	*secundum naturam* (according to nature)
Sn	*Stannum* (tin)
S/N	serial number; signal / noise (ratio)
SN	saddle nose; secretory nerve; senior; sensory nerve; serial number; sexual neurosis; somatic nerve; spinal nerve; spoon nail; student nurse; superficial necrosis; super-natural; suprasternal notch; surgical neck
SNAP	sensory nerve action potential
SNB	scalene node biopsy
SNHL	sensori-neural hearing loss
SNM	Society of Nuclear Medicine
SNN	stab-nuclear neutrophil
SNOP	Systematized Nomenclature of Pathology
s.n.p.	*signa nomine proporio* (label with the proper name)
SNP	Saturday night paralysis; sodium-nitro-prusside
SNR	signal-to-noise ratio
SNRT	sinus node recovery time
SNS	sympathetic nervous system
s.n.v.	*si non valeat* (if it is not enough)
s.o.	*scatula originalis* (original package)

SO	salpingo-oophorectomy; sense organ; sex organ; stitches out; subtotal operation; superior oblique; superior olive; sutures out; sympathetic ophthalmia
SO_2	sulfur-dioxide
SOA	spirit of ammonia; swelling of the ankles
SOAE	spontaneous oto-acoustic emission
SOAMCA	superficial occipital artery to middle cerebral artery
SOAP	Subjective, Objective, Assessment, Plan
SOB	shortness of breath
SOBW	shortness of breath with exertion
soc.	social; society
SOC	sequential-type oral contraceptive; spirit of camphor; stretching of contractures
SOCA	study of ocular complications of AIDS
SOD	stabilization of disease; super-oxide-dismutase
SODAS	Spheroidal Oral Drug Absorption System
SOE	salpingo-ovariectomy; spasm of esophagus
sol.	*solubilis* (soluble); *solutio* (solution)
SOL	space-occupying lesion
soln.	solution
solv.	*solve* (dissolve)
SOLVD	studies of the left ventricular dysfunction
SOM	secretory otitis media; serous otitis media; spirit of mustard
SOMI	sternal-occipital-mandibular immobilization
SOMIB	sternal-occipital-mandibular immobilization brace
Sono.	sonoencephalogram; sonogram; sonography; sonometer
SOP	Standard Operating Procedure
s.o.s.	only one dose; *si opus sit* (if it is needed; if necessary)
SOS	softening of stomach (gastromalacia)
SOW	staff of Wrisberg
s.p.	*sine prole* (without issue); single pole
sp.	special; *specialis* (specialist); species; specific; specimen; sperm; spermatid; spine; *spiritus* (spirit); spleen; spoon
S/P	status post; status posted; surgical procedure
SP	saccharum purificatum (pure white sugar); sacrum to pubis; shunt procedure; sinus pause; skin potential; sleeping pill; sleeping pills; speaker; specialist; status post; status posted; suicide precautions; steady potential; summating potential; supra-pubic; symphysis pubis; systolic pressure
2SP	transport medium (used for mycoplasma isolation)

SPA	single photon absorptiometry; supra-pubic aspiration
SPAI	steroid protein activity index
spat.	*spatula* (blade; spatula)
SPBI	serum protein-bound iodine
SPC	saturated phosphatidylcholine concentration
SPCA	serum prothrombin conversion accelerator; Society for the Prevention of Cruelty to Animals
SPCC	Society for the Prevention of Cruelty to Children
SPCT	simultaneous prism and cover test
SPE	serum protein electrophoresis
spec.	special; *specialis* (specialist); specific; specification; specimen; spectroscopy; speculum
spect.	spectroscopy
SPECT	single photon emission computed tomography; single positron emission computed tomography
SPEM	smooth pursuit eye movements
SPEP	serum protein electro-phoresis
SPF	specific pathogen free; sun protection factor
sp. fl.	spinal fluid
sp. gr.	specific gravity
sph.	spherical; spherical lens; sphingosine
SPH	secondary pulmonary hemosiderosis
SPHM	spectro-pyr-helio-meter
sp. ht.	specific heat
SPI	serum precipitable iodine
SPIA	solid phase immuno-assay
spir.	*spiritus* (spirit)
spis.	*spissus* (dried)
SPISA	solid phase immuno-sorbent assay
SPK	speaker; superficial punctuate keratitis
SPL	sound pressure level; spool
SPMG	stereo-photo-micro-graph
S/P-O	status post-operative
SPOOL	simultaneous peripheral operation on line
SPORE	Specialized Programs of Research Excellence
SPP	supra-pubic prostatectomy
SPRINT	Special Psychiatric Rapid Intervention Team
SPS	sodium-polyanethol-sulfonate; standards of physiological sleep; sulfite-polymyxin-sulfadiazine; superior petrosal sinus
SPSB	seclusio pupillae siderosis bulbi
spt.	*spiritus* (spirit)
SPTI	systolic pressure time index

SPV	single patient visit
sq.	*sequentia* (following; sequential); square
SQ	square; subcutaneous (injection)
sq. cm.	square centimeter (square centimetre)
SQUID	Superconducting Quantum Interference Device
sr.	steradian
Sr	senior; sister; Strontium
S&R	smooth and rough
SR	secretion rate; sedimentation rate; senior; sensitivity response; side rails; sigma reaction; single room; sinus rhythm; sister; skin resistance; stimulation ratio; superior rectus; surgery room; sustained release; swallowing reflex; system review; systemic resistance
SRBC	sheep red blood cell
SRC	sedimented red cell; sheep red cell
SRF	skin reactive factor; somatotropin releasing factor; split renal function; sub-retinal fluid
SRFA	slow-reacting factor of anaphylaxis
SRH	somatotropin-releasing hormone; stigmas of recent hemorrhage
SRIF	somatotropin-releasing inhibiting factor
SRM	Standard Reference Materials
S.R.N.	State Registered Nurse (of Britain and Wales)
sRNA	soluble ribo-nucleic acid
SRNV	sub-retinal neo-vascularization
SROM	spontaneous rupture of membrane
SRS	slow-reacting substance
SRS-A	slow-reacting substance of anaphylaxis
SRT	sedimentation rate test; speech reception threshold
SRV-1	simian retro-virus type 1
SRV-2	simian retro-virus type 2
SRY	sex-determining region Y
s̄ s̄	*semis* (one-half)
s/s	signs and symptoms; swish and swallow
ss.	*semis* (one-half)
S&S	signs and symptoms; swish and swallow
SS	saber shin; saline solution; saliva sample; Salmonella Schottmülleri; Salmonella-Shigella; salpingo-; salpingostomy; salpingoscope; saturated solution; Sézary syndrome; single side; single-sided; single source; single-stranded; sleeping sickness; soap-suds; somato-statin; straight sinus; super-saturated; synchronized sleep; systemic sclerosis

SSA	salicyl-salicylic acid; skin sensitizing antibody; Social Security Administration
SSAT	salicyl-sulfonic acid test
SSAV	simian sarcoma-associated virus
SSc	systemic sclerosis
SSC	similia similibus curantur
SSCER	somato-sensory cortically evoked response
SSD	source to skin distance
ssDNA	single-stranded deoxyribo-nucleic acid
SSE	soap-suds enema
SSEP	somato-sensory evoked potential
SSER	somato-sensory evoked response; smooth-surfaced endoplasmic reticulum
SSI	Social Security Income
SSKI	saturated solution of kalium-iodide (saturated solution of potassium-iodide)
SSL	second stage of labor
SSM	sulfapyridine-sodium-monohydrate; superficial spreading melanoma
SSN	Social Security Number
SSNHL	sudden sensori-neural hearing loss
SSPE	subacute sclerosing pan-encephalitis
ssRNA	single-stranded ribo-nucleic acid
s.s.s.	*stratum super stratum* (layer upon layer)
SSS	scalded skin syndrome; sick sinus syndrome; specific soluble substance; sterile saline soak; subclavian steal syndrome; super-saturated solution
SSSS	staphylococcal scalded skin syndrome
SSTZ	succinyl-sulfa-thia-zole
SSU	sterile supply unit
s.s.v.	*sub signo veneni* (under a poison label)
SSV	simian sarcoma virus; strabismus sursum vergens
s.t.	*sumat talem* (take one such)
st.	stand; station; *stet* (let it stand); *stetem* (let them stand); stitch; stomach; stone; straight; street
ST	*Salmonella typhimurium; Salmonella typhosa;* sedimentation time; serving time; sick-time; skin test; slight trace; smokeless tobacco; sore throat; spinal tap; stable toxin; standard time; standardized test; station; sterno-thyroid; stress test; stroke; sub-talar; sub-total; surface tension; survival time
S.T.37	hexylresorcinol (proprietary germicide and disinfectant)

STA	serum thrombotic accelerator; standard tube agglutination; station; superficial temporal artery
stab.	stabbed; stabilization; stabilizer
STA-MCA	superficial temporal artery — middle cerebral artery
Staph.	*Staphylococcus*
stat.	*statim* (immediately)
STATS	statistics
STc	sinus tachy-cardia
STC	soft tissue calcification
STCLV	simian T-cell leukemia virus
STD	sexually transmitted disease; skin test dose; skin-tumor distance; standard test dose; standard
STEAM	Streptonigrin, Thioguanine, Endoxan, Actinomycin D, Mitomycin C
STEL	short-term exposure limit
stg.	storage
STGC	syncytial trophoblastic giant cell
STH	somato-tropic hormone
STI	systolic time interval
STJ	sub-talar joint
STLI	sub-total lymphoid irradiation
STM	Streptomycin; short-term memory
STND	standard
STOC	sequential-type oral contraceptive
STOP	Swedish treatment of older people
STP	standard temperature and pressure
STPD	standard temperature and pressure — dry
STR	simple tumor removal; soft tissue rheumatism
Strep.	*Streptococcus*
STRs	superficial tendon reflexes
STS	serological test for syphilis
STSG	split-thickness skin graft
STT	scapho-trapezio-trapezoid; serial thrombin time
STTI	systemic tension-time index
STU	skin test unit
STV	simian T-virus
STVA	sub-total villose atrophy
STZ	Strep-to-zocin
SU	saccharum ustum (burnt sugar; caramel); Sunday
SUA	serum uric acid
sub.	*subinde* (frequently); substitute; subtract; subtraction
subcu.	subcutaneous

SUBG	Skene's urethral and Bartholin's glands
subin.	*subinde* (frequently)
subj.	subject
sub q	subcutaneous
suc.	*succus* (juice)
SUD	sudden unexpected death; sudden unexplained death
SUDS	sudden unexplained death syndrome
SUID	sudden unexplained infant death
SUIDS	sudden unexplained infant death syndrome
sum.	*sumat* (let him/her take); *sume* (take); *sumendum* (to be taken)
sum. tal	*sumat talem* (take one such)
Sun.	Sunday
SUN	serum urea nitrogen; Sunday
sup.	superior; *supervisus* (supervisor; having looked over)
supp.	*suppositoria* (suppository)
sur.	surgery; surgical
surg.	surgery; surgical
SUS	stained urinary sediment
susp.	*suspensio* (a hanging; suspension)
SUUD	sudden unexpected unexplained death
s.v.	*spiritus vini* (alcoholic spirit)
SV	Salk vaccine; simian virus; snake venon; stroke volume; subclavian vein; supra-vital
SV-40	simian virus 40 (simian vacuolating virus 40)
SVA	supra-ventricular activity
SVAS	supra-valvular aortic stenosis
SVB	supra-ventricular beats
SVBG	saphenous vein bypass graft
SVC	service; simultaneous ventilation compression; slow vital capacity; superior vena cava
SVC-CPR	simultaneous ventilation compression — cardiopulmonary resuscitation
SVCG	spatial vector-cardio-gram
SVC-RPA	superior vena cava — right pulmonary artery
SVCS	superior vena cava syndrome
SVD	Saint Vitus' dance; spontaneous vaginal delivery; spontaneous vertex delivery
SVF	*Staphylococcus viridis flavescens*
SVG	saphenous vein graft
SVI	stroke volume index
SVM	syncytial vascular membrane

SVO$_2$	mixed venous oxygen saturation
s.v.p.	*si vires permittant* (if the strength will permit)
SVPB	supra-ventricular premature beat
SVPTc	supra-ventricular paroxysmal tachy-cardia
s.v.r.	*spiritus vini rectificatus* (alcohol; rectified spirit of wine)
SVR	stroke volume ratio; supra-ventricular rhythm; systemic vascular resistance
SVRI	systemic vascular resistance index
s.v.t.	*spiritus vini tenuis* (proof spirit)
SVTa	supra-ventricular tachy-arrhythmia
SVTc	supra-ventricular tachy-cardia
Sv. unit	Sievert unit (a unit of gamma-ray dose)
s.v.v.	*spiritus vini vitis* (brandy)
SW	salt water; sea-water; short-wave; silk-worm; sleep walking; slow wave; spiral wound; stab wound; stroke work; switch
SWD	short-wave diathermy
SWGS	silk-worm gut suture
SWI	stroke work index
SWS	slow-wave sleep
Sx	sign; signs; symptom; symptoms
Sy.	syphilis; syrup
SYI	seven-year itch (scabies)
sym.	symbol; symmetrical; symmetry; symptom; symptoms
sync.	synchronization; synchronize
syr.	*syrupus* (sirup; syrup)
sys.	syssarcosis; systasis; system; systematic; systemoid; systole
syst.	systasis; system; systematic; systemoid; systole
syzy.	syzygiology; syzygium; syzygy
Sz.	seizure; Strepto-zocin

～ T ～

TCβ	throat culture — beta strep
t	tablespoon; teaspoon; temporal; tertiary; tight; time; ton; true
T	absolute temperature; kinetic energy; tablespoon; Taenia; tail; tall; tape; taste; tea; tear; tears; teaspoon; teeth; telephone; temperature; temporal; tense; tera- (= 10^{12}); terminal; tesla; testis; thorax; Threonine; throat; Thymidine; Thymine; tight; time; tissue; tocopherol; tolerance; ton; tongue; tooth; torque; transform; transmittance; transverse; treatment; Treponema; Trichophyton; true; Trypanosoma; tumor
$T°$	temperature
T^+	increased intraocular tension
$T-$	decreased intraocular tension
$t_{1/2}$	half-life; half-time
T_1	tricuspid valve closure
T_3	tri-iodothyronine
T_4	thyroxine
T1	first thoracic vertebra; longitudinal relaxation time; tumor 1
T2	second thoracic vertebra; transverse relaxation time; tumor 2
T3	tumor 3
T4	tumor 4
T 13-15	trisomy 13-15 — chromosomal abnormality
T 17-18	trisomy 17-18 — severe deformity and mental retardation
T 21	Down's syndrome (mongolism)
T-1824	Evans blue
T_h	temperature of hypothalamus
t_m	temperature — midpoint
T_m	temperature — melting
T_{max}	time — maximum concentration
T_{mg}	maximal tubular reabsorption of glucose
T_s	temperature — set-point
Ta	Tantalum

T&A	tonsillectomy and adenoidectomy
TA	alkaline tuberculin; axillary temperature; tarsal amputation; tarsal arches; Teaching Assistant; thenal aspect; therapeutic abortion; titratable acid; toxin-antitoxin; tropical abscess; tumor antigen
TAA	thoracic aortic aneurysm; thyroid auto-antibody; transfusion-associated AIDS; tumor-associated antibody; tumor-associated antigen
TAAb	teichoic acid anti-body
TA-AIDS	transfusion-associated acquired immuno-deficiency syndrome
TAANA	The American Association of Nurse Attorneys
tab.	*tabella* (tablet)
TAb	therapeutic abortion
TAB	therapeutic abortion
tabs.	tablets
TAB-vac.	typhoid-paratyphoid A and B vaccine
TAC	Tetracaine, Adrenalin, Cocaine; total abdominal colectomy
tach.	tachometer; tachycardia
tachy.	tachycardia
TAD	Thioguanine, Ara-C, Daunorubicin; thoracic asphyxiant dystrophy; transient acantholytic dermatosis
TADAC	Therapeutic Abortion, Dilation, Aspiration, Curettage
TAF	tissue angiogenic factor; toxoid-antitoxoid flocculus; trypsin aldehyde fuchsin; tumor angiogenic factor
TAH	total abdominal hysterectomy
TAH-BSO	total abdominal hysterectomy with bilateral salpingo-oophorectomy
tal.	*tales* (such a one); *talia* (such a one); *talis* (such a one)
TAL	thymic alympho-plasia
TAM	Tamoxifen; toxoid antitoxoid mixture
TAMI	thrombolysis and angioplasty in myocardial infarction
TANI	total axial node irradiation
TAO	thrombo-angiitis obliterans; tri-acetyl-oleandomycin (Troleandomycin)
Tap.	Tapazole
TAPVC	total anomalous pulmonary venous connection
TAPVD	total anomalous pulmonary venous drainage
TAPVR	total anomalous pulmonary venous return
TAR	thrombocytopenia absent radius; tissue-air ratio; treatment authorization request

TARA	total articular resurfacing arthroplasty; tumor-associated rejection antigen
TARS	thrombocytopenia absent radius syndrome
TASA	tumor-associated surface antigen
TAT	tetanus anti-toxin; Thematic Apperception Test; thromboplastin activation test; toxin-anti-toxin; turn-around time; tyrosine amino-transferase
tb.	table
t.b.	*tere bene* (rub well); tubercle bacillus; tuberculosis
Tb	Terbium; tubercle bacillus; tuberculin; tuberculosis
TB	temporal bone; terminal bronchiole; total base; total body; tracheo-bronchitis; tubercle bacillus; tuberculin; tuberculosis
TBA	tertiary butyl-acetate; testosterone-binding affinity; thio-barbituric acid; to be announced
TBD	total body density
TBE	tick-borne encephalitis; tuberculin bacillary emulsion
TBF	total body fat
TB fever	tick-borne fever
TBG	thyroxine-binding globulin
TBGP	total blood granulocyte pool
TBH	total body hematocrit
TBI	thyroxine-binding index; total body irradiation
TBII	TSH-BII (thyroid-stimulating hormone binding inhibitory immunoglobulin)
T. bili.	total bilirubin
TBK	total body kalium (total body potassium)
TBL	table
TBLC	term-birth living child
TBM	tuberculosis meningitis
TBP	Bithionol; thyroxine-binding protein; tick-bite paralysis
TBPA	thyroxine-binding pre-albumin
TbRD	tuberculosis respiratory disease
tbs.	tablespoon; tablespoonful
TBS	total body solute; tri-bromo-salicylanilide
TBSA	total body surface area
tbsp.	tablespoon; tablespoonful
TBT	tracheo-bronchial toilet
TBUA	thio-barbit-uric acid
TBV	total blood volume
TBW	total body water; total body weight
TBx	whole body irradiation
Tc	one billion cycles; Technetium; tetanic contraction

T&C	turn and cough; type and crossmatch
TC	tauro-cholate; technical component; temperature compensation; temporary carrier; tetra-cycline; thenar cleft; thermal capacity; thermal conductivity; throat culture; tissue culture; total cholesterol; total culture; total cystectomy; totally cured; trans-cobalamin; tuberculin contagious; tubo-curarine; tympanic cavity
TCA	transluminal coronary angioplasty; tri-carboxylic acid; trichlor-acetic acid
TCAD	tri-cylic anti-depressent
TC-ALL	thymus cell acute lymphoblastic leukemia
TCAP	Triazinate, Cytoxan, Adriamycin, Platinol
TCAR	thymus cell antigen receptor
TCB	throat culture — beta strep; total cardiopulmonary bypass; total color blindness
TCBS	thiosulfate citrate bile salts
TCC	transitional cell carcinoma; tri-chloro-carbanilide
TCD	thermal conductivity detector; tissue culture dose
TCD_{50}	tissue culture dose — 50%
TCDD	tetra-chloro-dibenzo-dioxin
TCE	tri-chloro-ethylene
T cell	thymus-derived cell
T-cell	thymus-derived cell
TCF	total coronary flow
TCG	tele-cardio-gram; tele-cardio-graphy; time compensation gain; time-controlled gain
TCGF	thymus cell growth factor
TCH	total circulating hormone
TCi	tetra-Curie
TCI	transient cerebral ischemia
TCID	tissue culture infective dose
$TCID_{50}$	tissue culture infective dose — 50%
TCIE	transient cerebral ischemic episode
TCL	tendo calcaneus lengthening
TCM	tissue culture media; Traditional Chinese Medicine
TCMA	trans-cortical motor aphasia
TCMI	thymus cell-mediated immunity
TCMIF	tumor cell migration inhibition factor
TCN	tetra-cycline
TCNB	Tecnazene
TCNS	trans-cutaneous nerve stimulator
TCO	total contact orthosis

TCP	tele-cardio-phone; tri-calcium phosphate; tri-cresyl phosphate; tumor control probability
TCPB	total cardio-pulmonary bypass
TcPCO$_2$	trans-cutaneous carbon dioxide pressure; trans-cutaneous carbon dioxide tension
TcPO$_2$	trans-cutaneous oxygen pressure; trans-cutaneous oxygen tension
tcRNA	translation control ribo-nucleic acid
TCSA	tetra-chloro-salicyl-anilide
TCT	thrombin clotting time; theca cell tumor (thecoma)
t.d.	*tempori dextro* (to the right temple)
TD	differentiated teratoma; temporary disability; tetanus-diphtheria; thoracic duct; through drainage; thymus-dependent; tolerance dose; tone deafness; torsion dystonia; toxic delirium; transverse diameter; treatment discontinued
TD$_{50}$	toxic dose — median
TD/5/5	tolerance dose — minimum
TD/50/5	tolerance dose — maximum
T-DA	TSH-DA (thyroid-stimulating hormone displacing antibody)
TDD	Telecommunication Device for the Deaf; thoracic duct drainage
TDE	tetrachloro-diphenyl-ethane
TDEE	total daily energy expenditure
TDF	thoracic duct fistula; thoracic duct flow; time dose factor; tumor dose fractionation
TDG	toko-dynamo-graph
TDI	toluene di-isocyanate; total dose infusion
TDL	thoracic duct lymph
TDM	therapeutic drug monitoring; toko-dynamo-meter; tour de maître (method)
TDN	total digestible nutrients
tDNA	transfer deoxyribo-nucleic acid
TDP	thermal death point; thoracic duct pressure
TDPA	tera-decanoyl-phorbol acetate
t.d.s.	*ter die sumendum* (to be taken 3 times a day)
TDT	thermal death time; tone decay test; tumor doubling time
Te	Tellurium; tetanus
TE	threshold energy; tissue-equivalent; total estrogen; toxic encephalitis; tracheo-esophageal

223

TEA	tetra-ethyl acid; tetra-ethyl-ammonium
TEAC	tetra-ethyl-ammonium chloride
TEAE-C	tri-ethyl-amino-ethyl cellulose
TEBG	testosterone estradiol-binding globulin
T&EC	trauma and emergency center
TECG	transesophageal echo-cardio-graphy
tech.	technical; technician; technology
TED	Tasks of Emotional Development; threshold erythema dose; thrombo-embolic disease
TEDD	total end-diastolic diameter
TEE	total energy expenditure; tyrosine-ethyl-ester
TEECG	trans-esophageal echo-cardio-graphy
TEF	thermic effect of food; tracheo-esophageal fistula
$Teff_{1/2}$	tumor effective half-life
TEG	telero-entgeno-graphy; thrombo-elasto-gram
TEIBQ	tri-ethylene-imino-benzo-quinone
TEL	telephone
tele.	telemetry; telepathy; telephone
TEM	transmission electron microscope; tri-ethylene-melamine
TEMP	temperature; temporary
TEMW	thermic effect of muscular work
TEN	toxic epidermal necrolysis
TENS	transcutaneous electrical nerve stimulation
TEP	thrombo-endo-phlebectomy; tracheal esophageal puncture
TEPA	tri-ethylene-phosphor-amide
TEPP	tetra-ethyl-pyro-phosphate
ter.	*tere* (rub)
tert.	*tertiarius* (tertiary)
TES	transcutaneous electrical stimulation
TESD	total end-systolic diameter
TET	treadmill exercise test
TETD	tetra-ethyl-thiuram-disulfide
TEV	talipes equino-varus
TEW	thermic effect of work
TF	tactile fremitus; thymol flocculation; toxic fume; transfer factor; transfer function; tuberculin filtrate; tubular fluid
TFA	total fatty acids
TFCC	triangular fibro-cartilage complex
TFE	tetra-fluoro-ethylene
Tfr.	transfer
TFS	testicular feminization syndrome

TFT	thyroid function tests; tight finger-tip; tri-fluoro-thyronidine (Trifluridine)
TF test	tuning-fork test
Tg	Thioguanine
TG	tendon graft; thyro-globulin; toxic goiter; tri-glycerides
TGA	thyro-globulin antibodies; transient global amnesia; transposition of great arteries
TGAR	total graft area rejected
TGES	transmissible gastro-enteritis of swine
TGF	therapeutic gain factor; transforming growth factor
TGFa	transforming growth factor a
TGFA	tri-glyceride fatty acid
TGFb	transforming growth factor b
TGT	thromboplastin generation test; thromboplastin generation time
TGV	thoracic gas volume; transposition of great vessels
Th	thigh; thoracic; Thorium; Thursday
TH	thigh; thoracic; Thursday; thyroid hormone
ThA	thigh amputation
THA	total hip arthroplasty; total hydroxy-apatite; transient hemisphere attack
THAM	tris-hydroxymethyl-amino-methane (Tromethamine)
THBR	thyroid hormone-binding ratio
THC	tetra-hydro-cannabinol (hashish; marijuana); tetra-hydro-cortisone; trans-hepatic cholangiogram
THCG	trans-hepatic cholangio-gram
THDC	tetra-hydro-deoxy-corticosterone
TH disease	thyroid heart disease
Theo.	Theocin; Theolix; Theophylline
THF	tetra-hydro-folate; tetra-hydro-furan
THFA	tetra-hydro-folic acid
THP	total hydroxy-proline
THR	threonine; Thursday; total hip replacement;
thru	through
THUM	Tamm-Horsfall urinary mucoprotein
Thur.	Thursday
Thurs.	Thursday
THz	tera-Hertz
Ti	Titanium
TI	thoracic index; through illumination; time in; time interval; tincture of iodine; total input; total ion; transverse inlet; tricuspid incompetence; tricuspid insufficiency

TIA	transient ischemic attack
TIBC	total iron-binding capacity
TIBD	tetrahydro-imidazo-benzo-diazepinone
TIC	trypsin inhibitory capacity
TI cell	Türk's irritation cell
t.i.d.	*ter in die* (three times a day)
TID	titrated initial dose
TIE	transient ischemic episode
TIF	tumor inhibitory factor
TIG	tetanus immune globulin
TIIV	trivalent inactivated influenza vaccine
TIL	tumor infiltrating lymphocytes; Türk's irritation leukocyte
TIMI	thrombolysis in myocardial infarction
t.i.n.	*ter in nocte* (3 times a night)
TIN	tubular interstitial nephropathy
tinc.	*tinctura* (tincture)
TIP	tincture of iodine poisoning
TIS	tumor in situ
TISS	Therapeutic Intervention Scoring System
TIT	Treponema immobilization test; tri-iodo-thyronine
TIVC	thoracic inferior vena cava
TJ	tendon jerk; toxic jaundice; triceps jerk; trochoid joint
TJR	total joint replacement
TK	thymidine kinase; traumatic keratitis; true knot
TKA	trans-ketolase activity
TKDG	to-ko-dynamo-graph
TKDM	to-ko-dynamo-meter
TKO	to keep open
TKR	total knee replacement
Tl	Thallium
TL	temporal lobe; thermo-luminescence; total lipids; total loss; toxic lesion; trial of labor; triangular lamella; tubal ligation; tuperculoid leprosy
TLA	thymus leukemia antigen
TLAG	trans-lumbar aorto-gram
TLAP	trans-luminal angio-plasty
TLC	tender loving care; thin-layer chromatography; total lung capacity; total lung compliance; total lymphocyte count
TLCS	thin-layer chromatography screen
TLD	thermal luminescent dosimeter; tumor lethal dose
TL Disease	Toulouse-Lautrec disease

TLE	thin-layer electrophoresis
TLG	tarsal lacrimal glands; tele-radio-graphy
TLH	total laparoscopic hysterectomy
TLI	thymidine labelling index; total lymphoid irradiation
TLP	tubo-ligamentary pregnancy
TLSO	thoracic lumbo-sacral orthosis
TLV	threshold limit value; total lung volume
Tm	Thulium
TM	technical manual; tectorial membrane; temporal mandibular; trademark; transcendental meditation; tremolo massage; tropical medicine; tympanic membrane
TMA	Tooth's muscular atrophy; tri-methoxy-amphetamine
TMAb	thyroid microsomal anti-body
TMB	transient monocular blindness
TMD	temporal mandibular disorder
TMF	thymocyte mitogenic factor
TMI	trans-mandibular implant
TMJ	temporo-mandibular joint
TMJD	temporo-mandibular joint dysfunction
TMJI	temporo-mandibular joint inflammation
TMJS	temporo-mandibular joint syndrome
TML	tetra-methyl lead
TMM	Thayer-Martin medium
TMN	tumor-node metastasis
TMP	trans-membrane pressure; trimethoxyphenyl-methyl-pyrimidinediamine (Trimethoprim)
TMP-SMX	Trimethoprim — Sulfamethoxazole
TMR	tissue maximum ratio
TMST	tread-mill stress test
TMT	tarso-meta-tarsal; Thiram
TMTD	tetra-methyl-thiuram-disulfide (Thiram)
TMV	tobacco mosaic virus
Tn	normal intraocular tension; Thoron
TN	tension; total needs; totally neutral; transfusion nephritis; trifacial neuralgia; trigeminal neuralgia; tubal nephritis
TNF	tumor necrosis factor
tng.	training
TNG	tri-nitro-glycerin
TNI	total nodal irradiation
TNM	tumor, nodes, metastasis
TNMR	tritium nuclear magnetic resonance
TNP	tri-nitro-phenyl

227

TNS	transcutaneous nerve stimulator
TNT	tri-nitro-toluene
TNTC	too numerous to count
TNZ	thermo-neutral zone
t.o.	turn over
TO	telephone order; time out; tincture of opium; total output; total oxygen; tuberculin (original); tubo-ovarian
TOA	tubo-ovarian abscess
TOC	test of cure
TOCP	tri-ortho-cresyl-phosphate
TOC syn.	thoracic outlet compression syndrome
TOD	target-object distance
TOEI	tissue oxygen extraction index
TOG	tension of gases
TOL	trial of labor
TOMHS	treatment of mild hypertension study
tomo.	tomogram; tomography
tomos	tomograms
top.	topically
TOP	termination of pregnancy; tincture of opium; toxemia of pregnancy; tubo-ovarian pregnancy
TOPS	Take Off Pounds Sensibly (name of an organization)
TOPV	trivalent oral poliovirus vaccine
TORCH	Toxoplasmosis, Other infections, Rubella, Cytomegalovirus infection, Herpes simplex
TORP	total ossicular reconstructive prosthesis
TOS	thoracic outlet syndrome
TOU	tumor of uterus
TOX	toxicity; toxicoderma; toxicology; toxicomania; toxicophobia
TP	testosterone propionate (male hormone); threshold potential; total protein; Trendelenburg position; *Treponema pallidum*; tri-phosphate; Tryptophan; tubal pregnancy; tube precipitin; tuberculin precipitation
t-PA	tissue plasminogen
TPA	tissue plasminogen activator; total parenteral alimentation; *Treponema pallidum* agglutination
TPBF	total pulmonary blood flow
TPC	total procto-colectomy
TPCCF	*Treponema pallidum* cryolysis complement fixation
TPCF	*Treponema pallidum* complement fixation
TPD	two-point discrimination
TPE	total protected environment

TPH	thymus persistens hyperplastica; transplacental hemorrhage
TPHA	*Treponema pallidum* hemagglutination assay
TPI	*Treponema pallidum* immobilization; *Treponema pallidum* isomerase; triose phosphate isomerase
TPIA	*Treponema pallidum* immobilization adherence; *Treponema pallidum* immune adherence
TPIT	*Treponema pallidum* immobilization test
TPM	temporary pace-maker; tri-phenyl-methane
TPN	total parenteral nutrition; triorthocresyl phosphate neuropathy; triphospho-pyridine-nucleotide
TPP	thiamine pyro-phosphate; trans-pulmonary pressure
TPPN	total peripheral parenteral nutrition; tri-phospho-pyridine nucleotide
TPR	temperature, pulse, respiration; testosterone production rate; total peripheral resistance; total pulmonary resistance
TPRI	total pulmonary resistance index
TPS	two-point sensibility; Trypsin (Parenzymoil)
TPSS	tumor poly-saccharide substance
TPT	*Treponema pallidum* test; typhoid para-typhoid (vaccine)
TPTI	thyro-para-thyro-idectomy
TPTZ	tri-pyridyl-tria-zine
TPVR	total peripheral vascular resistance
TQ	tocopherol-quinone; triple quartan
tr.	*tinctura* (tincture); treatment
TR	tetrazolium reduction; total reaction; total resistance; total response; trace; transfer rate; tricuspid regurgitation; Trypsin; tuberculin residue; tubular reabsorption
trach.	tracheal; tracheography; tracheoscopy; tracheostomy
TR-AIDS	transfusion related acquired immuno-deficiency syndrome
TRAMF	transverse rectus abdominis musculocutaneous flap
trans.	transaldolase; transfer; transformer; transistor; translate; translation; transport
TRAP	tartarate-resistant acid phosphatase
TRBF	total renal blood flow
TRBHC	trans-rectal biopsy of hypercholeic cancer
TRC	tanned red cells; total ridge count
TRDNB	transient respiratory distress of the newborn
TRE	true radiation emission
TRF	thymus-replacing factor; thyrotropin-releasing factor
TRFC	total rosette-forming cell
TRG	tele-roentgeno-graphy; tele-röntgeno-graphy

TRH	thyrotropin-releasing hormone
TRI	tetrazolium reduction inhibition
TRIA	thyroid radio-isotope assay
T$_2$-RIA	di-iodothyronine radio-immuno-assay
T$_3$-RIA	tri-iodothyronine radio-immuno-assay
T$_4$-RIA	thyroxine radio-immuno-assay
trid.	*triduum* (3 days)
trig.	triglycerides; trigonometry; trigger
TRIS	Trisamine (Tromethamine); tris buffer
trit.	*tritura* (grind; triturate)
tRNA	transfer ribo-nucleic acid
TRNG	tetracycline resistant *Neisseria gonorrhoeae*; training
Trp	Tryptophan
TRP	tubular reabsorption of phosphate
TRS	triaxial reference system; tumor reduction surgery; tumor reductive surgery
trt.	treatment
TRU	turbidity reducing unit
T$_3$RU	tri-iodothyronine resin uptake
TRUS	trans-rectal ultra-sound
TRUSG	trans-rectal ultra-sono-graphy
Try	Tryptophan
t.s.	*tempori sinistro* (to the left temple)
TS	temperature sensitive; test solution; thoracic surgery; threshold stimulus; tinea sycosis; tongue-swallowing; trans-sexual; transient sound; tricuspid stenosis; tropical sprue
TSA	total shoulder arthroplasty; trypticase soy agar; tuberculin skin anergy; tumor-specific antigen
TSB	trypticase soy broth
TSC	technetium sulfur colloid; thio-semi-carbizide
TSc-1	tuberous sclerosis type 1
TSc-2	tuberous sclerosis type 2
TSD	target-skin distance; Tay-Sachs disease
TSE	testicular self-examination; tri-sodium-edetate
TSF	thyroid-stimulating factor; triceps skin-fold
TSH	thyroid-stimulating hormone
TSH-BII	thyroid-stimulating hormone binding inhibitory immuno-globulin
TSH-DA	thyroid-stimulating hormone displacing antibody
TSH-RF	thyroid-stimulating hormone releasing factor
TSI	thyroid-stimulating immunoglobulin; triple-sugar iron
TSLS	toxic shock-like syndrome

TSM	*therapia sterilisans magna*
tsp.	teaspoon; teaspoonful
TSP	total serum protein; tri-sodium-phosphate; tropical spastic paraparesis
TSPAP	total serum prostatic acid phosphatase
T-spine	thoracic spine
TSR	thyroid to serum ratio
TSS	toxic shock syndrome
TSS-T1	toxic shock syndrome — toxin 1
TST	tumor skin test; two-step test
TSTA	tumor-specific transplantation antigens
TS test	two-step test
TSY	trypticase soy yeast
T&T	tone and turgor
TT	tablet triturates; teratoid tumor; test tube; tetanus toxoid; Tetrazol; thrombin time; thymol turbidity; tilt table; toilet training; tongue-tie; toxic tetanus; trans-thoracic; traumatic tetanus; tuberculin tested
TT$_4$	total thyroxine
TTA	tuberculin-type allergy
TTAD	tetra-cyclic anti-depressant
TTAP	threaded titanium acetabular prosthesis
TTC	telec-tro-cardiogram; triphenyl-tetrazolium-chloride
TTCG	telec-tro-cardio-gram
TTD	tissue tolerance dose
TT-ECG	trans-thoracic echo-cardio-graphy
TTEM	topo-therm-esthesio-meter
TTI	tension-time index
TTL	transistor-transistor logic
TTNB	transient tachypnea of the new-born
TTP	thrombotic thrombocytopenic purpura
TTPA	triethylene-thio-phosphor-amide (Tespamin; Tifosyl)
TTR	thermal tolerance ratio
TTS	temporary threshold shift; tuberculin-type allergy
TTT	tensor tympanic tendon; tolbutamide tolerance test
TTY	tele-typewriter
t.u.	toxic unit; tuberculin unit
Tu.	Tuesday
TU	Thio-uracil; toxic unit; tuberculin unit; tumor of uterus;
T$_3$U	tri-iodothyronine uptake
Tue.	Tuesday
Tues.	Tuesday

TUG	total urinary gonadotropin
TUL	total uterine length
TUP	tubo-uterine pregnancy
TUR	trans-urethral resection
TURB	trans-urethral resection of bladder
TURBT	trans-urethral resection of bladder tumor
TURP	trans-urethral resection of prostate
tus.	*tussis* (a cough)
TV	tele-vision; tidal volume; trial visit; Trichomonous vaginitis; triple vaccine; tuberculin volutin; tubo-vaginal; tubular vision; tunnel vision; typhoid vaccine
TVAT	true visual acuity test
TVC	timed vital capacity; total volume capacity; trans-vaginal cone; triple voiding capacity
TVD	triple vessel disease
TVDALV	triple vessel disease with abnormal left ventricle
TVF	tactile vocal fremitus
TVH	total vaginal hysterectomy
TVP	tricuspid valve prolapse
TVPM	trans-venous pace-maker
TVR	tonic vibration index; total vascular vibration; tricuspid valve replacement
TVT	*tunica vaginalis testis*
TVU	total volume urine
TW	tap water; total water; total weight; tunnel wound
TWD	total white and differential count
TWE	tap water enema
TWL	transepidermal water loss
TWX	teletype-writer exchange service
Tx	therapy; transplant; treatment;
TX	primary tumor cannot be accessed; thrombo-xane; traction
ty.	typhoid; typhus
typh.	typhoid; typhus
tyr.	tyrosine
tyro.	tyrosinaemia; tyrosine; tyrosinemia; tyrosinosis; tyrosinuria
Ty. sol.	Tyrode solution
TZ	tuberculin zymoplastiche; transition zone
TzT	Tzank test

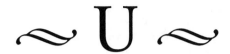

U

u	unified atomic mass unit; ulna-incomplete
U	international unit of enzyme activity; ulna-complete; unit; university; unknown; upper; uracil; Uranium; urgent; uridine; *urina* (urine); uterine
U/A	urinalysis (urine + analysis)
UA	umbilical artery; un-aggregated; uric acid; urinalysis (urine + analysis); uterine aspiration
UAC	umbilical artery catheter
UAO	upper airway obstruction
UAP	utero-abdominal pregnancy
UBB	ultimo-branchial body
UBBC	unsaturated B_{12} binding capacity
UBF	uterine blood flow
UBG	uro-bilino-gen
U&C	usual and customary
UC	ulcerative colitis; ulcus cancrosum; ulcus cruris; un-changed; unilocular cyst; upper case; urea clearance; uremic convulsion; urethral catheterization; uterine cast; uterine contractions; uterine cough
UCAMP	urinary cycle adenosine mono-phosphate
UCC	ulnar carpal complex; United Cancer Council
UCD	usual childhood disease
UCG	ultrasonic cardio-gram; urinary chorionic gonadotropin
UCHD	usual child-hood disease
UC/I	urethral catheter in; urinary catheter in
UCL	ulnar collateral ligament
UC/O	urethral catheter out; urinary catheter out
UCP	urinary copro-porphyrin
UCP/21	hexahydro-2, 7-dithio-1, 3, 6-thiadiazepine (etem)
UCPA	United Cerebral Palsy Association
UCR	un-conditioned reflex; un-conditioned response; usual, customary, and reasonable
UCS	un-conditioned stimulus; un-conscious; ureter-cysto-scope
UCTS	undifferentiated connective tissue syndrome
u.d.	*ut dictum* (as directed)

UD	urethral discharge
UDM	unit dose medication
UDP	uridine diphosphate
UDPG	uridine di-phosphate glucose
UDPGA	uridine di-phospho-glucuronic acid
UDPGal	uridine di-phospho-galactose
UDPGlc	uridine di-phospho-glucose
UDPGT	uridine di-phospho-glycyronyl transferase
UDPT	uridine di-phosphoglycyronyl transferase
UE	uncinate epilepsy; upper extremity; uricolytic enzyme
UES	upper esophageal sphincter
UF	ultra-filtrate; ultra-filtration; ultra-fine
UFA	unsterified fatty acids
UG	under-graduate; urethral glands; uro-genital; utero-gestation;utero-graphy
UGD	uro-genital diaphragm
UGFNAB	ultrasound-guided fine needle aspiration biopsy
UGI	upper gastro-intestinal (series)
UGIS	upper gastro-intestinal series
UGIT	upper gastro-intestinal tract
UGS	uro-genital sinus
ugt.	urgent
UH	upper high
UHCAN	Universal Health Care Action Network
UHF	ultra-high frequency
UHMWPE	ultra-high molecular weight poly-ethylene
UI	universal infantilism; urinous infiltration; uroporphyrin isomerase
UIBC	unsaturated iron-binding capacity
UIE	urine immuno-electrophoresis
UIEP	urine immuno-electro-phoresis
UIF	undegraded insulin factor
UIP	usual interstitial pneumonia; usual interstitial pneumonitis
UIQ	upper inner quadrant
UK	United Kingdom (England); un-known; uro-kinase
U&L	upper and lower
UL	ultra-low; undifferentiated lymphoma; un-listed; upper link; upper lobe
ULP	ultra-low profile
ULQ	upper left quadrant
ult.	ultimate; *ultime* (lastly)
UM	unmarried; unstriated muscle; uracil mustard

umb.	*umbilicus* (navel)
UME	uveo-meningo-encephalitis
UMLS	unified medical language system
UMN	upper motor neuron
UMP	uridine mono-phosphate
UN	ulnar nerve; umbilical notch; United Nations; urea nitrogen
unc.	*unctus* (smeared)
UNESCO	United Nations Educational, Scientific, and Cultural Organization
ung.	*unguentum* (ointment)
UNICEF	United Nations International Children's Emergency Fund
univ.	universal; university
UNK	unknown
UNRRA	United Nations Relief and Rehabilitation Organization
U/O	urinary output
UO	unknown origin; un-official; urethral orifice; urinary output
UOP	utero-ovarian pregnancy
UOQ	upper outer quadrant
UOV	utero-ovarian varicocele
u.p.	*ultimum praescriptus* (the last ordered; the last prescribed)
U/P	urine / plasma (ratio)
UP	unknown pressure; un-pack; uretero-pelvic; uro-porphyrin; urticaria papulosa; uterus parvicollis
UPA	utero-placental apoplexy
UPE	urine protein electrophoresis
UPEP	urine protein electro-phoresis
UPF	uveo-parotid fever
UPG	uro-porphyrino-gen
UPI	uretero-placental insufficiency
UPIN	unique physician identification number
UPJ	uretero-pelvic joint; uretero-pelvic junction
UPP	urethral pressure profile
UPPP	uvulo-palato-pharyngo-plasty
UQ	upper quadrant
ur.	uracil; *urina* (urine); urinalysis
U/R	unconditioned response; urgent reply
UR	unconditioned response; upper respiratory; urgent reply; urine; utilization review
ura.	uracil

URAC	Utilization Review Accreditation Commission
urd.	uridine
URD	upper respiratory disease
urg.	urgent
URI	upper respiratory infection
URO	urology
urol.	urology
URQ	upper right quadrant
URT	upper respiratory tract
URTI	upper respiratory tract infection
U/S	ultra-sound
US	ultra-sound; un-sweet; urinary sediments; urinary stammering; urinary stuttering; urinary system; urogenital sinus
USA	ultra-sonic atomizer
USAEC	United States Atomic Energy Commission
USAN	United States Adopted Names
USB	upper sternal border
USCI	United States Catheter Instruments
USD	United States Dispensary
USDA	United States Department of Agriculture
USG	utero-salpingo-graphy
USI	urinary stress incontinence
USN	ultra-sonic nebulizer
USP	United States Pharmacopeia
USPHS	United States Public Health Services
USR	unheated serum reagin
USRT	unheated serum reagin test
ust.	*ustus* (burnt)
usu.	usual
ut.	*uterus* (uterus)
UTBG	unbound thyroxine-binding globulin
utd.	*ut dictum* (as directed)
UTD	up-to-date
utend.	*utendus* (to be used)
UTG	utero-tubal gestation
UTI	urinary tract infection
UTP	uridine tri-phosphate
UTS	Ullrich-Turner syndrome (male Turner's syndrome)
UU	urine urobilinogen; utricle of the urethra
UUN	urine urea nitrogen
UV	ultra-violet; umbilical vein; urinary volume
UVA	ulcus vulvae acutum; ultra-violet A

UVB	ultra-violet B (sunlight)
UVBI	ultra-violet blood irradiation
UVC	ultra-violet C; umbilical venous catheter
UVEB	unifocal ventricular ectopic beat
UVEO	oveoparotid fever
UVGI	ultra-violet germicidal irradiation
UVJ	uretero-vesical junction
UVL	ultra-violet light
UVR	ultra-violet radiation
UVRT	ultra-violet radiation therapy
uvu.	uvulotomy; uvulotume; uvulotome (uvulatome)

$\sim V \sim$

$\bar{v}$	mixed venous
$\dot{v}$	gas flow
v.	*vel* (or); *vena* (vein); *vice* (in the place); *vide* (see)
V	vacuum; vagina; valine; valve; Vanadium; vector; vegetable; vein; velocity; venous; ventilation; ventricle; vibration; Vibrio; video; vision; voice; void; volt; voltage; volume; vomiting
V_1	chest lead 1: 4th intercostal space at the right sternal border
V_2	chest lead 2: 4th intercostal space at the left sternal border
V_3	chest lead 3: equidistant between V_2 and V_4
V_4	chest lead 4: 5th intercostal space at left of midclavicular line
V_5	chest lead 5: anterior axillary line
V_6	chest lead 6: mid-axillary line
V_7	chest lead 7: posterior axillary line
V_8	chest lead 8: posterior scapular line
V_9	chest lead 9: left border of the spine
V_a	alveolar ventilation
V_A	alveolar volume
V_c	blood volume of the capillary bed
V_D	anatomical dead space
V_r	relaxation volume
V_T	tidal volume
VA	vacuum aspiration; ventricular arrest; ventriculo-atrial; vertebral artery; Veterans' Administration; Vincent's angina; vision acuity; visual acuity; visual aid; volt-ampere
VABCD	Vinblastine, Adriamycin, Bleomycin, CCNU, Dacarbazine
vac.	vacuum
VAC	vacuum; Vincristine, Actinomycin D, Cyclophosphamide
VACTERL	Vertebral, Anal, Cardiac, Tracheal, Esophageal, Renal, Limb

VAD	vascular access device; venous access device; ventricular assist device; Vincristine, Adriamycin, Dexamethasone
VAdC	Vincristine, Adriamycin, Cytoxan
VAFAC	Vincristine, Amethopterin, FU, Adriamycin, Cytoxan
vag.	*vagina* (vagina); vaginal
VAIPP	vaso-active intestinal poly-peptide
val.	valance; validate; valine; value
VALE	visual acuity left eye
VAMP	Vincristine, Actinomycin D, Methotrexate, Prednisone
VA-ODLP	visual acuity oculus dexter light perception
VA-OSLP	visual acuity oculus sinister laeva perception (with projection)
VAP	Velban, Actinomycin D, Platinol
VAPA	Vincristine, Adriamycin, Purinethol, Ara-C
var.	variable; variant; variety; various
VARE	visual acuity right eye
vasc.	vascular
VASC	Verbal Auditory Screen for Children
VAT	ventricular atrial (synchronous); ventricular activation time; Veterinary Aptitude / Admission Test
VATD	Vincristine, Ara-C, Thioguanine, Daunomycin
VATERR	Vertebral defects, Anal atresia, Tracheoesophageal fistula, Esophageal atresia, Radial and Renal anomalies
vasc.	vascular
VAV	VePesid, Adriamycin, Vincristine
Vb	Vinblastine (Velban)
VB	varolian bend; Velban, Bleomycin; ventricular bradycardia
VBA	Velban, BCNU, Adriamycin
VBACS	vaginal birth after caesarean (cesarean) section
VBAP	Vincristine, BCNU, Adriamycin, Prednisone
VBC	ventricular brady-cardia; vitiamin B complex
VBD	van Buren's disease; Velban, Bleomycin, DDP
VBG	venous blood gas; venous bypass graft
Vbl.	Vinblastine
VBM	Vinblastine, Bleomycin, Methotrexate
VBMCP	Vincristine, BCNU, Melphalan, Cytoxan, Prednisone
VBP	Vinblastine, Bleomycin, Platinol
VBS	Veronal (barbital) buffered saline
VBS:FBS	Veronal (barbital) buffered saline : fetal bovine serum (ratio)
VBS/FBS	Veronal (barbital) buffered saline / fetal bovine serum (ratio)

V/C	voltage / circulation (ratio)
VC	vas capillare; vena cava; ventilatory capacity; vital capacity; vocal cord; venereal collar
VCA	viral capsid antigen
VCAP	Vincristine, Cytoxan, Adriamycin, Prednisone
VCAP-III	VePesid, Cytoxan, Adriamycin, Platinol
VCB	ventricular capture beat
VCC	vaso-constrictor center
VCD	vocal cord dysfunction
VCF	Vincristine, Cytoxan, Fluorouracil
VCFS	velocity of circumferential fiber shortening
VCG	vector-cardio-gram; vector-cardio-graphy
VCMP	Vincristine, Cytoxan, Melphalan, Prednisone
VCP	Vincristine, Cytoxan, Prednisone
Vcr	Vincristine
VCR	video cassette recorder
VCS	vena cava superior
VCT	venous clotting time
VCUG	voiding cysto-urethro-gram
VD	vagrant's disease; vas deferens; venereal disease; void; voided; volume of distribution
VDA	venous digital angiogram; visual discriminatory acuity
VDAG	venous digital angio-gram
VDBR	volume of distribution of bili-rubin
VDDR	vitamin D-dependent rickets
VDEL	Venereal Disease Experimental Laboratory
VDF	ventricular diastolic fragmentation
VDG	venereal disease gonorrhea
VDH	valvular disease of heart; vascular disease of heart
VDL	visual detection level
VDP	Vincristine, Daunomycin, Prednisone
VDRL	Venereal Disease Research Laboratory
Vds.	Vindesine
VDS	venereal disease syphilis
VDU	video dsplay unit
VE	vaginal examination; ventricular ectopic; visual efficiency; volumic ejection
VEA	ventricular ectopic activity
VEBs	ventricular ectopic beats
VECP	visual evoked cortical potential
VEDP	ventricular end-diastolic pressure
VEE	Venezuelan equine encephalomyelitis
VEEV	Venezuelan equine encephalomyelitis virus

241

VEF	ventricular ejection fraction
VEGF	vascular endothelial growth factor
VENP	Vincristine, Endoxan, Natulan, Prednisone
VEP	visual evoked potential
VEPA	Vincristine, Endoxan, Prednisone, Adriamycin
ver.	verification; verify; version
VER	visual evoked response
VERP	ventricular effective refractory period
vert.	vertical
VES	Vespresin injection (Etoposide)
VESI	vesiculogram; vesiculography
vesic.	*vesicatorium* (a blister); *vesicula* (vesicule)
vesp.	*vesper* (evening)
VESV	vesicular exanthema of swine virus
VET	veteran
VF	ventricular fibrillation; ventricular fluid; ventricular flutter; visual field; vocal fremitus
VFP	ventricular filling pressure; ventricular fluid pressure
VG	vaginal hernia; ventricular gallop
VGD	Von Gierke's disease
VGH	very good health
VH	vaginal hysterectomy; venous hepatitis; viral hepatitis
VHD	valvular heart disease
VHDD	viral haematic (hematic) depressive disease
VHDLP	very high density lipo-protein
VHF	very high frequency
VHS	viral hemorrhagic septicaemia (septicemia)
v.i.	*vide infra* (see below)
VI	valgus index; viscosity index; volume indicator
VIA	virus inactivating agent
vib.	vibration
vic.	vicinity
VIEN	vaginal intra-epithelial neoplasia; vulval intra-epithelial neoplasia
VIF	virion infectivity factor
VIG	vaccinia immune globulin
vin.	*vinum* (wine)
VIP	vasoactive intestinal polypeptide; Velban, Isofamide, Platinol; very important person; voluntary interruption of pregnancy
VIPST	vasoactive intestinal polypeptide secreting tumor
vir.	*viride* (green); *viridis* (green)

VIS	vaginal irrigation smear
vis-à-vis	as compared with; face to face (opposite); in relation to
VISI	volar intercalated segmental instability
vit.	vital; vitalist; vitamer; vitamin; *vitellus* (yolk of an egg)
viz.	*videlicet* (namely)
VL	very large; very late; very little; very low
VLA	very late antigen
VLBW	very low birth weight
VLCD	very low-calorie diet
VLDLP	very low-density lipo-protein
VLED	Visible Light Emitting Diode
VLF	very low fat; very low frequency
VLIA	virus-like infectious agent
VLM	visceral larva migrans
VLNH	very low nucleus of hypothalamus
VLP	Vincristine, Leucogen, Prednisone
VLSI	Very Large Scale Integration
VM	ventricular muscle; volt-meter
VM-26	Teniposide
VMA	vanillyl-mandelic acid
VMAD	Vincristine, Methotrexate, Adriamycin, Dactinomycin
VMBC	Vincristine, Melphalan, BCNU, Cytoxan
VMC	vaso-motor center
VMCP	Vincristine, Melphalan, Cyclophosphamide, Prednisone
V.M.D.	*Veterinariae Medicinae Doctor* (Doctor of Veterinary Medicine)
V-16-MF	VePesid, Methotrexate, Fluorouracil
VMH	ventro-medial hypothalamus
V.M.N.	*vis medica'trix naturae* (the healing power of nature)
VM-26-PP	Teniposide, Procarbazine, Prednisone
VMR	vaso-motor rhinitis
VN	visiting nurse
VNA	Visiting Nurse Association
VNR	vitro-nectin receptor
$\dot{V}O_2$	volume of oxygen consumption
$\dot{V}O_{2max}$	maximum volume of oxygen consumption
VO_2	volume of oxygen uptake
VO_{2max}	maximum volume of oxygen consumption
VOR	vestibular ocular reflex
v.o.s.	*visio oculus sinister* (vision of left eye); *vitello ovi solutus* (dissolved in yolk)
v.o.u.	*visio oculus uterque* (each eye vision)

V&P	vagotomy and pyloroplasty; ventilation and perfusion
VP	variegate porphyria; veni-puncture venous pressure; ventricular pause; ventricular peritoneal; vice-president; Vincristine, Prednisone; Vindesine, Platinol
VP-16	VePesid (Etoposide)
VPB	Velban, Platinol, Bleomycin; ventricular premature beat
VPC	vapor-phase chromatography; ventricular premature complex; ventricular premature contraction; volume of packed cells
VPCG	vapor-phase chromato-graphy
VPD	ventricular premature depolarization
VPF	vascular permeability factor
VPI	vapor phase inhibitor
VPL	ventro-posterior lateral (fetus position); Vincristine, Prednisone, Leucogen
VPP	virus pneumonia of pigs
VP-16-P	VePesid, Platinol
VPRC	volume of packed red cells
VPS	valvular pulmonic stenosis; ventilation perfusion scan
VR	vagina resection; valve replacement; variable region; vascular resistance; venous return; ventilation ratio; vocal resonance; vocational rehabilitation
VRBC	volume of red blood cell
VRI	viral respiratory infection
VRNA	viral ribo-nucleic acid
VQ scan	ventilation quantitation imaging technique
v.s.	vibration-seconds; *vide supra* (see above)
vs.	*versus* (in contrast with; versus)
V.S.	Veterinary Surgeon
VS	ventricular septum; vital signs; volumetric solution
VSD	ventricular septal defect
VSFP	venous stop flow pressure
VSGP	variable surface glycoprotein
VSL	very serious list
VSN	vital signs normal
VSPFT	Vitalor screening pulmonary function test
VSS	vital signs stable
VSV	vesicular stomatitis virus
VSW	ventricular stroke work
V&T	volume and tension
VT	vacuum tube; vacuum tuberculin; variable time; venous thrombosis; voice tube

VTc	ventricular tachycardia
VTE	venous thrombo-embolism
VTR	video tape recorder
VU	volume unit
VUR	vesico-ureteral reflux
vv.	*venae* (veins)
v.v.	vice versa
v/v	volume of solute per volume of solvent
V&V	vulva and vagina
VV	varicose veins; viper venom; vulva and vagina
V_D / V_T	dead space / tidal volume (ratio)
VVI	ventricular demand inhibited
VVT	ventricular demand triggered
VW	vessel wall
VZ	varicella-zoster
VZIG	varicella-zoster immune globulin
VZV	varicella-zoster virus

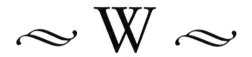

w/	with
w	with
W	wait; wash; water; watt; weak; Wednesday; week; weight; west; white; wide; widow; wife; window; Wolfram (tungsten); woman; work
W+	weakly positive
WA	well-arrange; when awake
WACH	wedge, adjustable, cushioned-heel (shoe)
WAIS	Wechsler Adult Intelligence Scale
WAPM	wandering atrial pace-maker
WAR	whole abdominal therapy
WART	whole abdominal radio-therapy
WAS	Wiskott-Aldrich syndrome
WASO	wake after sleep onset
WASP	World Association of Societies of Pathology
Wb	Weber
WB	waste-basket; water brush; water-bed; weight bearing; Western blot; wet brain; whole blood; whole body
WBAT	weight bearing as tolerated
WBC	well-baby care; white blood cell; white blood count; whole body counter
WBCD	white blood count and differential
WBC/hpf	white blood cell per high-power field
WBF	whole blood folate
WBGT	Wet Bulb Globe Temperature
WBGTI	Wet Bulb Globe Temperature Index
WBH	whole blood hematorit; whole body hyperpyrexia; whole body hyperthermia
WBHc	whole blood hemato-crit
WBHp	whole body hyper-pyrexia
WBHt	whole body hyperthermia
WBR	whole body radiation
WBS	whole body scan
WBV	Willow-brook virus

W/C	wheel-chair; white count
W.C.	toilet; water-closet (called rest-room in U.S.A.)
WC	walking cast; water-cure (hydrotherapy); waxy cast; wet cup; wheel-chair; white cell; white count; whooping cough; workman's compensation; wrist bones; writer's cramp
WCC	white cell casts; white cell count
WCD	Weber-Christian disease
WCG	Wrisberg's cardiac ganglion
WCHP	wood-chuck hepatitis virus
WD	well-developed; well-done; well-differentiated; wet dressing; wrist drop
W4D	Worth-four-dot (test)
WDHA	watery diarrhea with hypokalemic alkalosis
WDLL	well-differentiated lymphocytic lymphoma
WDWN	well-developed, well-nourished
We	Wednesday
WE	western encephalitis; western encephalomyelitis; wide excision
Wed.	Wednesday
WEE	western equine encephalitis; western equine encephalomyelitis
WEEV	western equine encephalitis virus; western equine encephalomyelitis virus
WEN	Westphal-Edinger nucleus
WEST	work evaluation systems technology
WF	white female
WFE	Williams flexion exercises
WFI	water for injection (pyrogen-free water)
WFR	Weil-Felix reaction
WGA	wheat germ agglutination
wgt.	weight
wh.	white
WH	watt-hour; writing hand
WHA	World Health Assembly
WHO	World Health Organization
WHR	waist-hip (circumference) ratio
WHS	Werdnig-Hoffmann syndrome
WHT	white
WHVP	wedged hepatic venous pressure
WI	water intoxication; water itch
WIA	wounded in action

WIC	women, infants, children
WISC	Wechsler Intelligence Scale for Children
wk.	weak; week; work
wks.	weeks
WL	waiting list; water low; wave-length; white leg; white line
WLE	wide local excision
WLF	whole lymphocytic fraction
WLT	water-load test
WM	white male; white mouse
WMA	World Medical Association
WMD	white-muscle disease
WMR	work metabolic rate
WMT	Weir Mitchell's treatment
WMX	whirlpool, massage, exercise
WN	well-nourished; wet-nurse
WNF	West Nile fever
WNL	within normal limits
WNV	West Nile virus
w/o	water in oil; without
WO	written order
WOB	water on brain (hydrocephalus)
WOE	white of egg; white of eye (conjunctiva)
WP	weakly positive; wedge pressure; wet pack; whirl-pool; white phosphorus; white precipitate
WPB	whirl-pool bath
WPM	words per minute
WPPSI	Wechsler Preschool Primary Scale of Intelligence
WPW	Wolf-Parkinson-White
WPWA	wedge pressure of pulmonary artery
WPWS	Wolf-Parkinson-White syndrome
wr.	wrist
WR	Wassermann reaction (a syphilis test); weakly reactive
Wr^a	Wright antigen
WRAT	Wide Range Achievement Test
WRC	washed red cells
WRE	whole ragweed extract
w.s.	water soluble; watt-seconds
wt.	weight (wiht in Old English)
WT	waiting time; waking time; walking time; walking typhoid; water temperature; wild type; wisdom teeth; writing table

WTFSBS	Wright's technique for staining blood smears
w/v	weight in volume; weight of solute per volume of solvent
WV	whispered voice; whole volume
w/w	weight in weight; weight of solute per weight of total solution

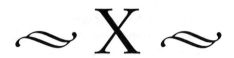

X

$\bar{x}$	except; mean
x	abscissa; mole fraction
X	cross; cross out; crossed out; decimal scale of potency; decimal scale of dilution; extra; times; magnification; multiply; reactance; respirations (anesthesia chart); unknown; xanthine; xanthosine
X_c	medical decision level
Xan.	xanthine
Xao.	xanthosine
XAT	Xylose Absorption Test
XB	xanthine bases
XC	xanthic calculus
XCG	excretory cysto-gram
XD	xanthoma diabeticorum; X-ray dermatitis
X-disease	bovine hyperkeratosis
XDP	xero-derma pigmentosum
Xe	Xenon
XECTG	Xenon-enhanced computed tomography
XESM	X-ray energy spectro-meter
XIP	X-ray in plaster
XL	extra large; extra long
XLDA	xylose lysine deoxycholate agar
XM	crossmatch; xanthoma multiplex
XMP	xanthosine-mono-phosphate
XMTR	transmitter
Xn	Christian
XOAN	X-linked ocular albinism Nettleship
XOD	xanthine-oxi-dase
XOP	X-ray out of plaster
XP	xanthoma palpebrarum; xeroderma pigmentosum; xylene poisoning
XR	xero-radiographic; xero-radiography; X-ray (x-ray); roentgen rays (röntgen rays)
XRF	X-ray fluorescence

XRFS	X-ray fluorescence spectrometry
XRG	xero-radiographic; xero-radiography
XRT	external radiation therapy; X-ray radiation treatment
XS	excess; excessive; xiphi-sternum; X-ray strain
XSA	cross-sectional area
X(T)	exotropia — intermittent
XT	exotropia; xanthoma tuberosum
XTAL	crystal
Xu	X-unit (x-unit)
XUG	excretory urogram
XX	normal female chromosome type
XX/XY	sex karyotypes
XY	normal male chromosome type
Xyl	xylene; xylose
Xyr.	xyrospasm
xys.	xysma; xyster

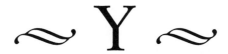

y	ordinate (in x-y axis); yard; year; yellow
Y	yard; year; yeast; yellow; yogurt (yoghurt); yolk; Yttrium
YAC	yeast artificial chromosome
YAG	yttrium aluminum (aluminium) garnet
Yb	Ytterbium
YB	year-book; yellow body (corpus luteum)
Y-chr.	Y chromosome
Y-crt.	Y cartilage
yd.	yard; yield
yds.	yards
YE	yellow; yellow enzyme
YF	yellow fat; yellow fever; Y-factor (Pyridoxine)
YFV	yellow fever vaccine
YHT	Young-Helmholtz theory
Y-lig.	Y ligament (ilio-femoral ligament)
y/o	year old
YO	year of; years old
YOA	year of accident
YOB	year of birth
YOM	year of marriage
YOPLL	year of potential life lost
YOS	year of surgery
YPLL	years of potential life lost
yr.	year; younger
YR	Young's rule (rule for calculating the dose of medicine)
yrbk	yearbook
yrs.	years
YS	yellow spot (macula flava; macula lutea); Yersin's serum; yolk sac; yolk stalk
YSC	yolk sac carcinoma
YT	youth
YV	yellow vision
YW	yellow wax

~ Z ~

z	zero; zone
Z′	increasing degree of contraction 1
Z″	increasing degree of contraction 2
Z	atomic number; carbobenzoxy; impedance; increasing degree of contraction; ionic charge number; zuckung (German word meaning contraction)
ZA	zinc acetate; zoster auricularis; zygomatic arch
ZAT	Zondek-Aschheim test
ZB	zygomatic bone
ZC	zinc-chloride
Z/D	zero defect
ZD	Z disk; zero defect
ZDV	zi-do-vudine
Z-E	Zollinger-Ellison
ZEEP	zero end-expiratory pressure
ZES	Zollinger-Ellison syndrome
ZFY	zinc finger Y
ZG	zoo-graft; zoo-grafting
ZIG	zoster immune globulin
ZIGV	zoster immune globulin vaccine
ZIP	zoster immune plasma
Z-lig.	Zinn's ligament
ZMAC	zygo-matico-auri-cularis
Zn	Zinc
ZNM	Ziehl-Neelsen method
$ZnSO_4$	zinc-sulfate
ZO	zinc ointment; zinc oxide; zoster ophthalmicus
ZOE	zinc-oxide eugenol
ZOL	zonule of Zinn
zool.	zoologist; zoology
Z-P	z-plasty
ZPG	zero population growth
Z-plasty	Z-Plastic relaxing operation
ZPP	zinc proto-porphyrin

Zr	Zirconium
ZR	zygomatic reflex
ZS	zinc salts; zinc-stearate; zinc-sulfate
ZSP	zinc salts poisoning
ZSR	zeta sedimentation rate; zeta stimulation rate
zyg.	zygapophysis; zygion; zygoma
ZYM	zymometer; zymoscope; zymosimeter
zz.	*zingiber* (ginger)
ZZ	zonule of Zinn

Appendix A
Common Medical Symbols

+	acid reaction; and; increase; increased; plus; positive; present; slight trace
++	moderate; trace
+++	increased; moderately active; moderately severe
++++	large amount; pronounced reaction; severe
−	absent; charge already made (bookkeeping abbreviation); decrease; decreased; minus; negative
(+)	significant
(-)	insignificant
±	plus or minus; positive or negative
(±)	possibly significant
×	cross out; times (used with a number)
× 1	once
× 2	twice
× 3	thrice
× 4	four times
1 ×	once
2 ×	twice
3 ×	thrice
4 ×	four times
#	number
:	is to; ratio symbol
/	divided by; division; of; per; ratio symbol
÷	divided by; division
=	equal
≠	not equal
‖	parallel
∞	infinity
Σ	summation
~	approximately
%	percent; percentage
∠	angle
⊥	perpendicular
∴	therefore
?	doubtful; questionable

>	greater than
<	less than
≥	greater than or equal to
≤	less than or equal to
↑	increased; up
↓	decreased; down
→	move to right; results in; yields
←	move to left
↔	two-way operation
∧	diastolic blood pressure
∨	systolic blood pressure
√	check; checked; observe for
*	birth
†	dead; death; died
∅	empty; no change
⊕̸	no balance due (bookkeeping abbreviation)
⊖	start of operation
⊗	end of operation
α	alpha particle
β	beta chain of hemoglobin; beta ray
Δ	change; prism diopter
Δt	time interval
ΔEF	ejection fraction response
γ	conductivity; gamma; Ig; photon; surface tension
γA	IgA
γBF	IgBF
γD	IgD
γE	IgE
γG	IgG
γM	IgM
ψ	pseudouridine; psychiatrist; psychologist
ε	electric field intensity; electromotive force; permittivity
η	efficiency; viscosity
κ	kaon
λ	wavelength
∧	lambda particle
μ	magnetic momentum; mass absorption coefficient; micro; micron; modulus; muon; permeability; population mean; the heavy chain of IgM; viscosity
μA	micro-ampere
μC	micro-Coulomb
μCi	micro-Curie
μEq.	micro-equivalent

μg	micro-gram
μl	micro-liter (micro-litre)
μL	micro-liter (micro-litre)
μm	micro-meter (micro-metre)
μM	micro-molar
μmg	micro-milli-gram
μmm	micro-milli-meter (micro-milli-metre)
μP	micro-processor
μR	micro-roentgen (micro-röntgen)
μsec	micro-second
μU	micro-unit
μV	micro-volt
μW	micro-watt
μμ	micro-micro- (pico-)
μμCi	micro-micro-Curie (pico-Curie)
μμg	micro-micro-gram (pico-gram)
ν	degrees of freedom; frequency; kinetic viscosity; neutrino; reluctivity
π	3.14159265......; osmotic pressure; pion; the ratio of diameter and circumference of a circle
Ξ	xi particle
ρ	correlation coefficient; density; electric charge density; mass density; resistivity; rho particle
σ	1/1000 of a second; conductivity; cross-section; standard deviation; surface tension
Σ	sigma particle; sigmoid; sigmoidoscopy
τ	mean life; torque; transmittance
φ	electric potential; file; luminous flux; magnetic flux
Ω	ohm; omega particle
¶	paragraph
§	numbered clause; section
@	at
$0.00	credit (bookkeeping abbreviation)
&	and
$\overline{a}$	before
Å	Angstrom
Ã	cumulated activity
$\overline{aa}$	of each
AΩA	Alpha Omega Alpha (an honorary society in U.S.A.)
A>B	air greater than bone
Ⓑ	both
B√	billing information posted
B>A	bone greater than air

259

B↑E	both upper extemities
B↓E	both lower extemities
BS↓	breath sounds diminished
c̄	with
/c̄	with
c̄c	with correction (eye-glasses)
c̄ / c	with correction (eye-glasses)
©	confidential (patient may be unaware); copyright
C₅	caesarean section (cesarean section)
°C	temperature degrees in Celsius
/d	per day
°F	temperature degrees in Fahrenheit
↑FOB	elevate foot of bed
Ⓗ	hypodermic
↑ICP	increased intra-cranial pressure
Ⓛ	left
L→R	left to right
mμ	milli-micron
mμCi	milli-micro-Curie
mμg	milli-micro-gram
Ⓜ	murmur
M+C	morphine and cocaine
Ⓝ	notified
p̄	after
®	registered; right
℞	*recipe* (dispense — used at the beginning of a prescription)
℞ₓ	*recipe* (dispense — used at the beginning of a prescription)
R√	receipt done
R↑E	right upper extremity
R↓E	right lower extremity
ren∠	renal angle
R→L	right to left
s̄	without
/ s̄	without
s̄c	without correction (eye-glasses)
s̄ / c	without correction (eye-glasses)
s̄s̄	one half
Ŝ	spatial vector in electrocardiology
tγ̇	shear time
T°	temperature

T+	increased intraocular tension
T-	decreased intraocular tension
$\bar{x}$	except
♂	male
♀	female
⚣	gay
⚢	lesbian

APPENDIX B
Greek Alphabet

Capital letter	Small letter	Pronunciation	English equivalent
A	α	alpha	a
B	β	beta	b
Γ	γ	gamma	g, n
Δ	δ	delta	d
E	ε	epsilon	e
Z	ζ	zeta	z
H	η	eta	e (e as in easy)
Θ	θ	theta	th
I	ι	iota	i
K	κ	kappa	k
Λ	λ	lamda	l
M	μ	mu	m
N	ν	nu	n
Ξ	ξ	xi	x
O	o	omicron	o
Π	π	pi	p
P	ρ	rho	r, rh
Σ	σ	sigma	s
T	τ	tau	t
Y	υ	upsilon	y, u
Φ	φ	phi	ph
X	χ	chi	ch
Ψ	ψ	psi	ps
Ω	ω	omega	o (o as in flow)

APPENDIX C
Common Cardinal Numerals

Name	Arabic	Roman
zero (cipher; naught)	0	...
one	1	I
two	2	II
three	3	III
four	4	IV
five	5	V
six	6	VI
seven	7	VII
eight	8	VIII
nine	9	IX
ten	10	X
eleven	11	XI
twelve	12	XII
thirteen	13	XIII
fourteen	14	XIV
fifteen	15	XV
sixteen	16	XVI
seventeen	17	XVII
eighteen	18	XVIII
nineteen	19	XIX
twenty	20	XX
thirty	30	XXX
forty	40	XL
fifty	50	L
sixty	60	LX
seventy	70	LXX
eighty	80	LXXX
ninety	90	XC
one hundred	100	C
two hundred	200	CC
three hundred	300	CCC
four hundred	400	CD
five hundred	500	D

Name	Arabic	Roman
six hundred	600	DC
seven hundred	700	DCC
eight hundred	800	DCCC
nine hundred	900	CM
one thousand	1000	M
two thousand	2000	MM
five thousand	5000	$\overline{V}$
ten thousand	10000	$\overline{X}$
one hundred thousand	100000	$\overline{C}$
one million	1000000	$\overline{M}$

Metric Weights and Measures

LENGTH

unit	abbreviation	equivalent
centimeter (centimetre)	cm	0.393 inch
decameter (decametre)	dam	32.81 feet = 393.7 inches
decimeter (decimetre)	dm	3.937 inches
dekameter (dekametre)	dam	32.81 feet = 393.7 inches
hectometer (hectometre)	hm	109.36 yards = 328.08 feet
kilometer (kilometre)	km	0.621 miles
meter (metre)	m	39.37 inches = 3.28 feet
millimeter (millimetre)	mm	0.039 inch

AREA

unit	abbreviation	equivalent
hectameter (hectametre; hectare)	ha	2.471 acres
square centimeter (square centimetre)	cm²; sq. cm	0.15499 square inch
square decimeter (square decimetre)	dm²; sq. dm	15.499 square inches
square dekameter (square dekametre)	dam²; sq. dek.	393.7 square inches
square kilometer (square kilometre)	km²; sq. km	0.386 square mile = 247.1 acres
square meter (square metre)	m²; sq. m	1549.9 square inches = 1.196 yards
square millimeter (square millimetre)	mm²; sq. mm	0.00155 square inch

LAND

unit	abbreviation	equivalent
are		119.6 square yards
centiare	cent.	1549.9 square inches
hectare (hectameter; hectametre)	sq. hec.	2.471 acres
square kilometer (square kilometre)	km²; sq. km	0.386 square mile = 247.1 acres

VOLUME

unit	abbreviation	equivalent
cubic centimeter (cubic centimetre)	c.c.; cm^3	0.06102 inch cubic
cubic decimeter (cubic decimetre)	c.d.	61.023 cubic inches = 0.0353 cubic foot
cubic meter (cubic metre)	c.m.; m^3	35.314 cubic feet = 1.308 cubic yards
stere	st.	35.314 cubic feet = 1.308 cubic yards

CAPACITY

unit	abbreviation	equivalent
centiliter (centilitre)	cl; cL	0.6 cubic inch = 0.338 fluid ounce
deciliter (decilitre)	dl; dL	61.02 cubic inches = 0.21 pint = 3.38 fluid ounces = 0.1057 liquid quart
dekaliter (dekalitre)	dal; daL	0.35 cubic foot = 2.64 gallons = 0.284 bushels
hectoliter (hectolitre)	hl; hL	3.53 cubic feet = 1.14 pecks = 26.418 gallons = 2.838 bushels
kiloliter (kilolitre)	kl; kL	1.307 cubic yards = 264.18 gallons = 35.315 cubic feet
liter (litre)	l; L	61.02 cubic inches = 1.057 liquid quarts = 0.908 dry quart
milliliter (millilitre)	ml; mL	0.06 cubic inch = 0.27 fluid dram

MASS & WEIGHT

unit	abbreviation	equivalent
centigram	cg	0.1543 grain = 0.000353 ounce (avoirdupois)
decigram	dg	1.543 grains
decagram (dekagram)	dag	0.3527 ounce = 154.323 grains
gram	g; gm	0.0352 ounce (avoirdupois) = 15.432 grains
hectogram	hg	3.574 ounces
kilogram	kg	2.2046 pounds
metric ton	Mt, t	1.1 tons = 2204.6 pounds
milligram	mg	0.01543 grain
myriagram	myg	22.046 pounds
quintal	q	220.46 pounds

COMMON WEIGHTS

Unit Scale	Grams	Grains
1 Kilogram	1000	15432.35
1 Hectogram	100	15432.23
1 Decagram	10	154.3235
1 Gram	1	15.43235
1 Decigram	0.1	1.543235
1 Centigram	0.01	0.1543235
1 Milligram	0.001	0.01543235

APPENDIX E
Common Decimal Factors

SI PREFIXES
(Measurement)

The following prefixes are used to indicate decimal multiples and submultiples of SI units.

Prefix	Symbol	Factor
tera	T	10^{12}
giga	G	10^{9}
mega	M	10^{6}
kilo	k	10^{3}
hecto	h	10^{2}
deka	da	10^{1}
deci	d	10^{-1}
centi	c	10^{-2}
milli	m	10^{-3}
micro	μ	10^{-6}
nano	n	10^{-9}
pico	p	10^{-12}
femto	f	10^{-15}
atto	a	10^{-18}